D1577846

How to
Heal Yourself
using
Hand Acupressure
(Hand Reflexology)

by Michael Blate

How to
Heal Yourself
using
Hand Acupressure
(Hand Reflexology)

by Michael Blate

FALKYNOR BOOKS
Davie, Florida

This book is presented as a catalog and primer of techniques and other information that have been in continuous use throughout the Oriental and Western world for many years. While these techniques and information utilize a natural system within the body, there are no claims made for their effectiveness, even when properly used. These techniques and information are not an alternative to proper medical care and treatment, nor are they intended to supersede or replace any standard, Western first aid, emergency or medical techniques.

Illustrated by Michael Blate and Laurie Blate

Cover design by Andrea Holly Gold

Copyright© 1982 by Michael Blate.
Published by Falkynor Books, Davie, FL
Library of Congress catalog card number:
ISBN: 0-916878-21-X

All rights reserved, which include the right to reproduce this book or portions thereof in any form whatsoever. For information, address Falkynor Books, P. O. Box 290057, Davie, FL 33314.

Library of Congress cataloging and publication data:
Blate, Michael, 1938-
    How to Heal Yourself Using Hand Acupressure (Hand Reflexology)
    Bibliography:

Printed in the U.S.A.

10 9 8 7 6 5 4 3

This book is for Joy.

"Of the twenty-four hours which comprise a day, use six for earning and spending, six for contemplation of God, six for sleep and six for service to others."

Sri Sathya Sai Baba

Other books you will enjoy and find useful by this author, published by Falkynor Books:

* A Way of Eating for Pleasure and Health
* First Aid Using Simple Remedies
* Five Minutes to Fitness with Acugenics
* (The) G-Jo Institute Manual of Medicinal Herbs
* (The) G-Jo Institute Manual of Vitamins and Minerals
* How to Beat Stress with Acugenics
* How to Enjoy Sex More with Acugenics
* How to Lose Weight Easily with Acugenics
* How to Relieve Arthritis with Acugenics
* How to Stop Smoking with Acugenics
* How to Heal Yourself using Foot Acupressure (Foot Reflexology)
* (The) Natural Healer's Acupressure Handbook, Volume I: Basic G-Jo
* (The) Natural Healer's Acupressure Handbook, Volume II: Advanced G-Jo.
* (The) Tao of Health: The Way of Total Well-Being

Any of these books may be purchased through your local bookstore, health food store or directly from the publisher.

Falkynor Books
Post Office Box 290057,
Davie, Florida 33314

CONTENTS

ACKNOWLEDGMENTS

The author wishes to thank and gratefully acknowledge the help and assistance of many members and friends of The G-Jo Institute. He is especially grateful to:

* Laurie Blate
* Al Fon
* Andrea Holly Gold
* Dick Knierim
* Sandy Pasquale
* Diane Ruby
* Barbara Sisson
* Jimmy Sullivan
* Sharon Tufaro
* Gail Watson
* Peggy Wells

For further information about the format and design of this book, please see the colophon (located on the last page).

WHAT IS THE G-JO INSTITUTE?

The G-Jo Institute is a not-for-profit natural health research and educational organization. It was informally organized in 1976 and incorporated in 1982. Its purpose is the development and dissemination of drugless "self-health" techniques.

G-Jo is a simplified form of acupuncture without needles (or "acupressure"). However, the scope of the G-Jo Institute has expanded far beyond its original purpose of the sharing of simple acupressure techniques.

It is our belief that it is the body-mind — and only the body-mind — which heals itself. For that reason, we now address ourselves to the entire spectrum of how to stimulate the innate self-healing mechanisms witihin the body-mind with simple, yet effective, self-health techniques from around the world.

For further information or catalogs about our publications, recordings, workshops and such, send a business-sized, self-addressed stamped envelope to:

THE G-JO INSTITUTE
DIVISION D
POST OFFICE BOX 8060
HOLLYWOOD, FLA. 33024
U.S.A.

HOW TO USE THIS MANUAL

1. Read the following information and familiarize yourself with the techniques described in this manual;

2. Look up your symptom or disorder in Section I (or, if you are not suffering any specific symptoms but wish to use hand acupressure as a general wellness and prevention technique, go immediately to step 4A);

3. Refer to those illustrated points detailed in Section II, suggested for that specific symptom you wish to treat. (Note: While most of the acupressure points have names that correspond to the symptom or bodily area each point controls, a few are simply referred to by a cross-reference listing — e.g., F18, A14, etc. These refer to unnamed points and are located by moving up or down the appropriate number line on the chart to the appropriate letter or horizontal line; this will correspond to the approximate location on your own hand);

4. Begin deeply pressing and "working" that approximate area on your own hand until you find one or several sensitive and tender spots that correspond to that area;

OR

4A. Deeply massage the entire hand until you discover all the tender spots — and then mark an "X" in the illustration of the hands that is found on page 110 (which may be photocopied, so as not to have to mark this book), for future reference and self-treatment;

5. Work the tender point(s) as deeply as you can manage for 30 seconds or less — they should become more tender (and may stay that way for up to several days) as self-treatment continues;

6. Rest for awhile afterwards;

7. Repeat self-treatment up to several times daily in the beginning of the process, but gradually reduce hand acupressure over the following period of several weeks;

8. Stop any obvious abuses (e.g., smoking, eating or drinking to excess, etc.) that may lead to — or aggravate — the problem...study as many natural health publications and techniques as you can... improve your diet...and take any other necessary steps to keep — or restore — pleasure, happiness and health to your life;

AVOID HAND PRESSURE IF:

...you are a pregnant woman (especially beyond the third month of pregnancy);
...you are weakened, seriously ill or are taking regular medication for serious health problems (e.g., cancer, diabetes, etc.);
...you are a chronic heart patient (especially one who wears a pacemaker or other artificial energy-regulating device).

OVERVIEW

Hand acupressure — sometimes called "hand reflexology" — is an ancient "self-health" technique that has been widely used throughout the Orient for thousands of years and which has become popular in the Western world since the late 1960s. It is an easy-to-perform method to restore health and wellness, or to bring yourself symptomatic relief. This technique may be used by anyone in normal health up to several times daily (see instructions at the beginning of this book).

Hand acupressure points are thought to have both a diagnostic and therapeutic value. If you have a specific symptom — say, a headache or low back pain — you may immediately turn to that specific symptom in Section I of this manual and discover the appropriate hand acupressure points to help relieve and "reverse" (heal) that symptom.

Or, you may simply work on your entire hand — pressing deeply until you discover tender spots — then refer to Section II until you find the illustrations of points which correspond to the tender areas you have discovered. These may give you insight as to the state of your internal organs and glands (each of these points is thought to be somehow "connected" to a so-called "reflex," which in turn leads to a specific bodily area, organ or gland).

These points should be stimulated bilaterally — that is, on both hands — unless otherwise stated. The information about — and the location of the actual site of — these points has been drawn from a number of sources. Even so, their location on the illustrations is approximate: The only true method for actually finding your own points is to press deeply — using up to 20 lbs. of pressure — until you contact a tender and sensitive "ouch point" in that approximate area of your own hand.

If you cannot find such a point in the approximate area, it usually means that you are either not pressing deeply enough, or the point is not going to be therapeutically effective. Nearly always, the most tender points are also the most effective for bringing relief and promoting healing. And for therapeutic purposes, use only points which are tender to the touch. When they are no longer tender, discontinue their use.

Avoid any acupressure point that lies beneath a scar, mole, wart, etc. Wait about four hours after taking drugs, medications, alcohol (or other intoxicants) before applying hand acupressure. Wait about half an hour after taking a hot bath, doing strenuous labor or exercise, or eating a heavy meal before applying this technique. Other than that, acupressure may by used at any time.

HOW HAND ACUPRESSURE WORKS

Hand acupressure is thought to work by affecting the flow of vital "life force" throughout the system. A complete healing network of energy-carrying channels is said to terminate in the hands. At one end of each channel is an organ, gland or other bodily area. At the other end — in the hand — is an acupressure point. Life force moves along these channels, like electricity, to and from its various "terminals."

When life force — which we may call "bioenergy" — moves either too quickly or slowly along the channels, the organ or other bodily part malfunctions; symptoms and suffering soon follow. When a useful acupressure point is "triggered" and stimulated, it appears to at least temporarily restore a more normal or balanced flow of bioenergy.

ABUSE CAUSES SUFFERING

The process of disease and suffering is complex, yet the cause of most disease may be summed up in one word: Abuse. We abuse ourselves in many ways — wrong foods and drink...unloving thoughts and emotions... work or home situations that are stress-filled and demeaning...the use of tobacco and/or recreational drugs — the list sometimes seems endless.

Surprisingly, most abuse is voluntary and self-inflicted. On one hand this reveals our own foolishness and self-destructive nature; yet on the other hand, this is a fortunate state of affairs — abuses which we inflict upon ourselves voluntarily can also be controlled, released or eliminated, if we so desire.

Neither acupressure — nor any other natural health technique — can be truly successful unless and until certain rules of healing are obeyed. These rules include the following:

1. To get well we must first want to get well (this is the cardinal rule of healing — no healing can occur unless and until we intend it to happen and commit ourselves fully to the process);

2. We must discover — then release — the self-abusive practices which keep us ill and suffering; to speed healing, it is wise to replace abusive practices with a better "healthstyle" — right diet, moderate pleasures and spiritual self-development being of key importance;

3. We must be diligent in our efforts. Most adult (chronic) suffering follows years of abuse, and what takes years to develop cannot be cured in a matter of days;

4. We must not become discouraged. The human body-mind is a powerful self-healing mechanism that is capable of "reversing" (healing) many of even the most grievous ailments... as long as the above rules are followed.

ABOUT "HEALING PHENOMENA"

Illness and suffering arise from abuses which are somehow "stashed" and stored within the various organs we are about to stimulate through hand acupressure. The results of these abuses may be thought of as "toxins" that will be purged from the system as the healing process continues.

It is not unusual for "healing phenomena" — brief periods of cleansing — to occur during the course of hand acupressure. This is a natural process — and a beneficial one — so it should be understood and appreciated.

Typical symptoms of cleansing include: Changes in bowel movements; headaches (especially at the beginning of self-therapy); digestive upsets; or similar ailments and malaise that might indicate "a flow of trash" being dumped into the system. Symptoms of cleansing might even include emotional distress (e.g., depression, bouts of anger, etc.). These symptoms — if they occur — should be mostly eliminated within several weeks of beginning hand acupressure.

However, unlike symptoms of illness, healing phenomena usually "feel right" — we do not sense that we are ill while "suffering" them... only cleansing ourselves.

NOTE TO READERS:

In the following pages, those words, acupressure points or references which are fully CAPITALIZED are considered to be the most important. Those words, points or references which are underlined are considered of next importance.

ALSO: Following some of the acupressure point names or numbers, you will find a question mark (?). This should be taken as the author's suggestion — neither confirmed nor denied by other published healers, teachers or writers in the field of acupressure — as to the most useful point(s) for the target symptom or bodily area. When the question mark precedes all acupressure points, this means the author has not had first-hand experience with that point or series of points for that symptom/bodily area, but his suggestion is based upon his understanding of the "Energy (acupuncture) Theory" and its applications.

SECTION I

SYMPTOMS, BODILY AREAS AND THE HAND ACUPRESSURE POINTS WHICH AFFECT THEM:

Abdomen, lower
Abdomen, upper
Acne
Addiction
Adrenal glands
Alcohol, problem with
Allergies, non-specific
Anemia
Angina pectoris
Ankle
Anus
Apex (top of head)
Apoplexy (stroke)
Appendicitis
Appetite control
Appetitie stimulation
Arm
Arthritis, minor
Asthma and asthmatic
    breathing, wheezing, etc.
Athlete's foot
Back, lower and/or upper
Baldness (alopecia)
Birth control
Bites, animal, human and insect

Bites, spider
Bladder, urinary
Bleeding gums
Boils, styes, carbuncles
Bones
Brain
Brainstem
Breasts
Breathing, difficult and labored
Bronchitis
Burns and scalds, including
    sunburn
Bursitis
Buttocks
Car sickness
Cataracts
"Charley horse"
Cheeks
Chest
Cirrhosis
Clavicle (collarbone)
Coccyx
Colds and influenza
Colic, intestinal
Colitis
Colon
Congestion, sinus or nasal
Conjunctivitis (pink eye)
Constipation (costiveness)
Corns and bunions
Coronary thrombosis
Cough
Cramps, menstrual
Cramps and spasms, muscular
Cystitis
Dandruff
Deafness (sudden, acute)

Dental work
Depression (mental, emotional)
Dermatitis
Diabetes (diabetes mellitus)
Diaphragm
Diarrhea
Diverticulitis, diverticulosis
Dizziness
Dreaming, excessive
Duodenum
Dysentery
Dyspepsia
Dyspnea
Ear
Eczema
Edema
Elbow (including "tennis
    elbow")
Endocrine glands
Epiglottis
Epilepsy and epileptic
    seizures
Esophagus
Eustachian tubes
Eye
Face
Fatigue
Fear control centers
Fertility
Fever control centers
Fingers
Fits
Flatulence
Flu
Foot
Forehead
Fractures

Frigidity (sexual)
Frostbite
Gallbladder
Gallstones
Gastritis (acid indigestion)
Gastrointestinal system
Genital weakness, pain, etc.
Genitourinary system
Gingivitis
Glands, swollen
Glaucoma
Gonorrhea
Gout
Hair
Hand
Hangover
Hay fever
Head
Headaches
Hearing difficulties
Heart
Heart attack, heart failure
Heatstroke
Heel
Hemorrhage (bleeding)
Hemorrhoids (piles)
Hepatitis
Hernia (rupture)
Herpes simplex virus II
Herpes zoster virus
High blood pressure
Hip
Hives and rash (urticaria)
Hoarseness
Hunger control centers
Hyperactivity
Hypertension (high blood
   pressure)

Hypoglycemia
Hysteria
Ileo-cecum
Impetigo and eczema
Impotency (sexual)
Indigestion
Infection
Inflammation
Influenza
Insomnia
Intestinal problems
Intoxication
Itching; itchy skin
Jaundice
Jaw, lower
Jaw, upper
Kidneys
Kidney stones
Knee
Laryngitis
Larynx
Leg
Leg cramps (at night)
Liver
Low blood sugar
Lumbago
Lungs
Lymph glands or nodes
Mastitis
Mastoid process
Menopause
Menstrual difficulties
Migraine
Mouth
Multiple sclerosis
Mumps
Muscles
Nasal congestion (catarrh)

Neck
Nephritis
Nerves
Nervousness
Neuralgia
Neurasthenia
Nightmares
Nose
Nosebleed (epistaxis)
Numbness
Occiput (back of head)
Ovaries
Pain control centers
Palate
Pancreas
Panic
Paralysis
Parasites, internal
Parathyroid glands
Parotid glands
Pelvis
Perineum
Periodontal problems
Peritonitis
Pharynx
Pineal gland
Pituitary gland
Pleurisy
Pneumonia
Prostate
Psoriasis
Rectum
Respiratory system
Retching
Rheumatism
Rhinitis
Scapula
Sciatica

Seasickness
Sexual drive
Sexual organs
Shingles
Shoulder
Sinusitis
Skin
Small intestine
Snoring
Solar plexus
Sores
Sore throat
Spasm, muscular
Spinal cord
Spleen
Sprains, muscular
Stomach
Stones, gallbladder
Stones, kidney or bladder
Strains, muscular
Styes
Sweating control centers
Swelling
Tachycardia, paroxysmal
Tennis elbow
Testicles, including crushed
    testicles
Tetanus (lockjaw)
Thigh
Throat
Thyroid (and parathyroid)
    gland
Tinnitus
Toes
Tongue
Tonsillitis
Tooth, teeth
Toothache

Tooth extraction, drilling,
    etc.
Torticollis (stiff neck)
Trachea
Travel sickness
"Traveler's diarrhea"
Trigeminal neuralgia
Ulcers, digestive
Ulcers, oral
Ulcers, skin
Ureters
Urethra
Urinary control centers
Uterus
Vaginitis
Varicose veins
Vertebrae, cervical
Vertebrae, lumbar
Vertebrae, sacral
Vertebrae, thoracic
Vertigo
Vitiligo
Vomiting and retching
Whiplash (neck injury)
Wrist

Hand Acupressure points found at the end of each symptom's description.

ABDOMEN, LOWER (also see: Appendicitis; Peritonitis; etc.):. The area between the navel and the pubic region. Organs found in this area include: The small intestine; colon (large intestine); urinary bladder; sexual/reproductive organs; etc. Consider the following:
1. Pain that occurs throughout the entire abdomen (lower and upper) that is not localized nor extreme (a simple "bellyache") is probably from wrong food, constipation, etc;
2. Pain that occurs first at/near the navel, then shifts to the lower right quarter of the abdomen may be appendicitis;
3. Pain that is severe, cramplike and comes/goes, plus recurrent vomiting, abdominal distention, being gas-bound and constipated may indicate complete or (if there is diarrhea) partial blockage of the small intestine (esp. if pain centers at/near navel and if you have had an abdominal operation in the past);
4. Pain below the navel that's not too severe and is accompanied by distention, with difficulty in passing gas as well as difficulty in moving bowels (passing small, frequent stools, if any) may indicate partial/complete blockage of the colon/large intestine;

5. If you are a woman suffering pain in the lower right or left quarters of the abdomen that is sudden, severe and often accompanied by nausea and vomiting, it may be due to problems in the ovary, especially a twisted ovarian cyst;

6. Severe pain in the lower abdomen that gradually moves upward to the right upper quarter and stomach, increasing in intensity without relief (and with abdomen becoming hard) may be a symptom of peritonitis;

7. Frequently recurring pain that is relieved by passing gas, stools and especially if also accompanied by nausea, diarrhea, headaches, etc., may indicate colitis, pre-colitis or irritable colon;

8. Any lump in the groin or navel area, with or without pain, may indicate a hernia;

9. There are a number of other possibilities — intestinal flu, allergic reactions, poisoning, etc. — which might be considered;

If symptoms are not relieved by the following techniques, do the following:

1. Try each of the other sections listed for the above symptoms (e.g., Appendicitis, Gastrointestinal system, etc.) that most closely matches your symptoms;

2. If you still get no relief, avoid all foods and take only small amounts of water (or ice chips);

3. Get medical attention immediately.

Hand points: Appendix; Colon (all); Ileo-cecum; etc.

ABDOMEN, UPPER (also see: Small intestine; Stomach; etc.): The area between the diaphragm and the navel.

Included in this central portion of the body are: The liver; gallbladder; stomach; spleen; pancreas; small intestine; kidneys; adrenals; etc.

Pain/discomfort in the upper abdomen may indicate:

-18-

1. Simple indigestion — especially if the symptoms include: Nausea; heartburn; distention; a feeling of fullness; belching and/or flatulence; or any other similar symptoms which develop during or after a meal;

2. Gallbladder disorder — especially if the discomfort is located in the upper right quarter of the abdomen;

3. Pancreatitis (or other disorders of the pancreas) — especially if there is severe pain centering at/near the stomach, but extending to the back and chest and relieved by sitting up;

4. Heart attack, heart failure — which, in the beginning stages, is confused by some people with acute indigestion, etc.

As with disorders of the lower abdomen, there are many possible causes of distress. Follow the same rules as for problems in that region (see Abdomen, Lower);

Hand points: Middle third of hand plus corresponding bodily parts.

ACNE (also see: Allergies, non-specific; Skin; etc.): Eruptions on the face, chest, back, etc. Acne is thought to arise from imbalance within the lungs, colon, kidneys and urinary bladder by traditional Oriental therapists. (Note: Acne tends to worsen during winter, to improve during summer, but excessively hot and/or humid weather may trigger an attack, as may the time just before, during and/or after menses).

Hand points: Lungs; Kidneys; plus corresponding bodily areas; Endocrine glands (use cautiously).

ADDICTION (to alcohol, drugs, tobacco, etc. — also see): Alcohol, problems associated with; INTOXICATION; etc.: Marked emotional or psychophysical dependence on a substance — usually destructive — which is beyond voluntary control. In traditional Oriental theory, dependency and addiction are considered disorders primarily of the spleen, pancreas and stomach ("Earth" organs).

Hand points: (?) Lungs; Liver; Stomach; Spleen; Pancreas.

ADRENAL GLANDS (also see: Endocrine glands; Hypoglycemia; Kidneys; etc.): Endocrine glands are found just above the kidneys; they are responsible for the production of adrenaline (epinephrine) and numerous other steroid hormones. Any self-treatment of these glands should be done with caution and restraint.
The adrenals are key glands in regulating bodily reactions to stress and fear; their malfunctioning may result in allergies, hypoglycemia, arthritis, asthma, etc.

Hand points: Adrenals; Endocrine glands; Kidneys.

ALCOHOL, PROBLEMS ASSOCIATED WITH (also see: Cirrhosis; INTOXICATION; etc.): Studies show that females have a much lower tolerance for alcohol than males.

Hand points: Hypothalamus (?); Endocrine glands; Liver; Spleen; Pancreas.

ALLERGIES, NON-SPECIFIC (also see: Other symptoms associated with allergies): A repeated bodily reaction upon exposure to an allergenic substance such as wool, feathers, etc.

"Unusual" or "hidden" symptoms of allergy may include: Insomnia; excessive perspiration; restlessness; increased sense of smell; depression; abnormal pulse and many other seemingly unrelated phenomena.

Allergies are generally not cured but rather are greatly reduced by proper "healthstyle." Each person has at least several foods/substances to which he is allergic. Food allergies, at least, appear to come in "degrees" (or "layers") so that after the most offensive abusive allergen is dropped or eliminated from the diet, the allergy(ies) next in "strength" begin exerting their influence. At the root of each allergy is thought to be the emotion of <u>fear</u> controlled by the kidneys and adrenal gland).

Hand points: Appendix; Ileo-cecum; Adrenals.

ANEMIA (iron-deficiency type): A deficiency of red blood cells that is difficult — perhaps dangerous — to self-diagnose. Because internal bleeding (or such blood disorders as leukemia) may be responsible for this symptom, seek medical advice if anemia is suspected.

Hand points: Liver; Thyroid; Intestine, small; Spleen; Colon (all); Endocrine glands.

ANGINA PECTORIS (also see: Chest; Heart; Heart attack, heart failure; Pain control centers etc.): Deep spasmodic pain often radiating to the left arm and shoulder. It is often triggered by an emotionally or physically taxing experience. Get medical help immediately. Except in emergency, no pressure point stimulation should be used when regular daily medication is being taken; also, except when professional help is not available, self-treatment of heart disorders should be avoided (angina is the pain associated with coronary heart disease).

Angina is characterized by a pain (usually) in the center of the chest which also triggers a sense of fear or foreboding — a sense of warning that commands the sufferer to immediately stop what he is doing.

Angina responds quickly to rest. If the pain continues for longer than 15 minutes after relaxing, the pain is probably not angina.

Hand points: Heart; Chest.

ANKLE (also see: Foot; Sprains, muscular; Strains, muscular; etc.): For any injury to this joint, quickly remove shoe and stocking, since swelling tends to be rapid.

Hand points: Ankle; Heel.

ANUS (also see: Colon; Gastrointestinal system; Hemorrhoids; Rectum; etc.): Lowest point of the rectum and termination of the alimentary canal. Common symptoms include: Hemorrhoids; prolapse (dropping or drooping of wall of colon through the anus); rectal itch; etc.

Possible causes of anal itch include: Rectal disorders (hemorrhoids, etc.); pinworms (or similar parasites); allergies; various diseases (e.g., diabetes, venereal herpes simplex virus, jaundice, uremia, etc.); infection from fecal matter; worms, internal parasites.

<u>Hand points</u>: Anus; Rectum; Prostate (females, also); Perineum.

APEX (top) of Head (also see: Head; etc.): For pain or other symptoms in this area.

<u>Hand points</u>: Brain; Head.

APOPLEXY (stroke): The result of a blood clot or hemorrhage to the brain or a major organ.
   While nearly all strokes are accompanied by some disability — usually paralysis, etc. — it is important to remember that much can be done to restore full/nearly full recovery. Aside from the following acupressure points, other "alternative" methods (such as acupuncture done with needles) are also available.

<u>Hand points</u>: Liver; Pituitary; A-18; C-21; D-22; E-22; F-20; F-22.

APPENDICITIS (also see: Abdomen, lower; etc.): An inflammation of the appendix, located below and slightly to the right of the navel. This may be a serious problem; there is the possibility of the appendix rupturing. <u>Get medical help immediately</u>.
   Many other problems may mimic appendicitis, such as: Stones/infection in the urinary tract (esp. in the ureter); ileitis; ovarian cyst in a female; etc.

<u>Hand points</u>: Appendix; Colon, ascending; <u>Forehead</u>.

APPETITE CONTROL: See HUNGER CONTROL.

APPETITE STIMULATION: To help improve and stimulate the desire and hunger for food. Chronic loss of appetite may produce anorexia nervosa, a potentially dangerous condition of self-starvation (common especially among weight-conscious women and those who have successfully lost a substantial amount of excess weight). Get professional help for this condition. Any pressure point stimulation should be gentle and brisk (vs. deep, goading triggering).

Hand points: (?) Digestion; Stomach; Liver; Gallbladder.

ARM (also see: Elbow; Hand; Shoulder): Including both the arm and armpit. There are several (potentially) serious problems that can happen to the arm. Among them are:
    1. Arterial blockage — characterized by: Sudden coldness, tingling and/or numbness developing in the arm, followed by severe pain; blue or mottled patches developing on the skin, etc.;
    2. Fracture — characterized by: Sudden, sharp pain, especially upon movement of the affected arm;
    3. Thrombophlebitis (clot lodged in a vein) — characterized by: Warming of the skin at/near affected site; swelling; deep (esp. sudden) aching pain; etc.
    4. Symptom of heart disease (e.g., angina pectoris), impending/progressing heart attack, etc. — especially if pain radiates down the left arm.
If you notice any of the above symptoms, get medical help immediately.

Other less serious problems may include: Strains; sprains of the elbow, wrist, shoulder; inflammation; etc.

Hand points: Arm; Occiput.

ARTHRITIS, MINOR (acute): A catchall name for a number of symptoms that manifest themselves primarily as inflammation of the joints; it is suffered mostly by women. There are numerous self-help techniques detailed in this author's book, HOW TO RELIEVE ARTHRITIS WITH ACUGENICS (available through The G-Jo Institute).

Hand points: Use points for affected bodily areas; also: Endocrine glands.

ASTHMA and ASTHMATIC BREATHING, WHEEZING, ETC. (also see: Dyspnea; Hysteria; etc.): Massive narrowing and constriction of the air passages in the throat. Its symptoms include coughing, wheezing, panic, etc. Get medical help immediately.
    Most studies agree that an asthmatic's parents are an important root in the disorder — either overly protective or too unconcerned. Any therapy should take this into consideration.

Hand points: Lungs; Adrenals; C-18; D-18.

ATHLETE'S FOOT (also see: Foot; Toes; etc.): A damp, itching rot between the toes. Associated with a kidney disorder arising from excess animal protein (e.g., meat, eggs, etc.), according to traditional Oriental acupressure therapists.

Hand points: Forehead.

BACK, LOWER and/or UPPER (also see: Lumbago; Pain control centers Sciatica; etc.): Backache — especially lower backache — is one of modern man's most common symptoms. "Common" low back pain is often as much a disorder of the abdominal (bulky, unsophisticated lower trunk) muscles as one of the lower back. Back pain may also result from a number of more serious disorders (e.g., kidney stones, etc.) — if symptoms persist, see your doctor.

Hand points: Vertebrae; Spinal cord; Coccyx; Waist; Leg.

BALDNESS (alopecia): Often caused by excess male hormones in system. Generally hair loss is normal, as is hair regeneration; life of a strand of hair is about three years. Imbalanced or malfunctioning liver and kidneys are considered the organs most responsible for hair loss. Where there is baldness in front, it may be a symptom of excess fruits, liquids or intestinal disorders; when baldness is mostly on top, excess animal protein; when baldness occurs in back, excess drugs or chemicals; when baldness occurs at temples, may indicate excess sweets, drugs.

Hand points: Thyroid; Head; Kidneys; Lungs — also: Briskly whisk all last knuckles (those just behind nails) and the nails back and forth across each other for about 30 seconds daily.

BIRTH CONTROL: There are a number of natural methods to promote or prevent pregnancy. However, they should only be used with discretion and only when willing to accept the consequences of failure. The various acupressure points that may be useful include:

Hand points: Stimulate Kidneys to increase fertility.

BITES, ANIMAL, HUMAN AND INSECT: If you are bitten by a wild creature, there is a possibility of rabies, especially if the bite is from a skunk, squirrel, raccoon or other small mammal. Try capturing the animal alive for observation in captivity. Killing the animal is less desirable; but if done, keep the head refrigerated until it can be tested in a laboratory.

There are three possible states for a rabid animal to be in:
1. Furiously vicious, foaming at the mouth, etc.;
2. Sluggish-to-paralyzed;
3. Behaving "peculiarly" — that is, without normal fear of humans, aggressive behavior, daylight activity in ordinarily nocturnal creatures (e.g., bats, foxes, etc.).

Bites from animals in the above states call for immediate attention.

Hand points: Corresponding bodily area points.

BITES, SPIDER: Many spiders are somewhat poisonous, but the two most common truly poisonous spiders are the (female) black widow and the brown household (or brown recluse). Symptoms include pain, abdominal cramps, sometimes paralysis, tenderness, redness, and swelling around the bitten area. Get medical help immediately.

Hand points: Corresponding bodily area points.

BLADDER, URINARY (also see: STONES, KIDNEY OR BLADDER; Cystitis; Genitourinary system; Urinary control centers;): The organ of accumulation for urine. In traditional Oriental theory, this is considered one of the twelve principal organs and is paired with the kidneys. As such, it helps "control" fear, sexual drive, caution, etc. (For more in-depth techniques for healing this organ, see this author's THE NATURAL HEALER'S ACUPRESSURE HANDBOOK, VOLUME II.)

Hand points: Bladder (urinary); Kidneys.

BLEEDING GUMS: See GINGIVITIS.

BOILS, STYES, CARBUNCLES (also see: SKIN; "Sores"; etc.): Localized "staph" infections of varying degrees of severity. They are often found around the eyes (styes), neck, back, or buttocks. Often associated with disorders in the genitourinary system.

Hand points: Use corresponding bodily area points.

BONES (also see: Fractures; etc.): Bones are related to kidneys, according to Oriental therapists. Any bone disorders may also indicate kidney imbalances.

Hand points: Kidneys; Adrenals; corresponding bodily area points.

BRAIN (also see: Brainstem; Nerves; etc.): Primary portion of the central nervous system.

Hand points: Brain; Forehead; Head; Pituitary; Pineal.

BRAINSTEM (also see: BRAIN; etc.): Central part of the brain.

Hand points: Brain.

BREASTS: (also see: Mastitis; etc.): Intimately related to the stomach and/or liver in Oriental literature.

Hand points: Stomach; Chest.

BREATHING, Difficult and Labored: See DYSPNEA.

BRONCHITIS (also see: Chest; Cough; Respiratory system; Throat; etc.): An inflammation of the bronchial "tree" whose symptoms include fever, pains in the back and muscles, headache, etc.

Hand points: Adrenals; Colon; Lungs; C-18; D-18.

BURNS and SCALDS, including sunburn: There are different types of burns as well as degrees of severity:

a. Thermal (heat) burns: Immerse the area in a slush of freshwater ice and water, or let cold water flow from faucet onto burned area (up to 15 minutes);

b. Chemical burns: Flush chemicals from the tissue immediately;

c. Sunburn.

Minor (first-degree burns) cause redness and minor swelling to the affected site. More serious burns manifest blisters and additional swelling (second-degree) or leave the skin looking white or charred (third degree — the worst kind of burn). Third-degree burns may not be as painful as the less serious form because of underlying nerve damage. If a limb has been burned, keep it elevated. In more serious burns, shock is likely.

For more serious burns, drink plenty of water with a little salt and baking soda added to help replace the salty fluids of the body and reduce the possibility of shock. Do not apply ointments or pastes such as baking soda in the case of a severe burn; they will only have to be scraped off at a hospital or burn center. Get medical help immediately.

Hand points: Corresponding bodily area points.

BURSITIS (also see affected areas, such as Shoulder, etc.): An inflammation between moving joints. Immobilize the affected extremity (generally the arm or shoulder).

Hand points: Shoulder; or corresponding bodily area points.

BUTTOCKS (also see: Hip; etc.):

Hand points: Hip; Coccyx; Perineum; Waist; Kidneys; Sciatic nerve.

CAR SICKNESS: See SEASICKNESS; etc.

CATARACTS (also see: Eyes; etc.): Partial or complete opacity of the eye lens or its capsule. Often related to diabetes, excess galactose (from milk), fatty acid intolerance, irradiation, drugs, etc. May be related a liver disorder, according to Oriental therapists.

Hand points: Eye; Liver; Gallbladder.

"CHARLEY HORSE": See CRAMPS and SPASMS, MUSCULAR; LEG; STRAINS, MUSCULAR.

CHEEKS (also see: Face; Head; Mouth; etc.):

Hand points: Head; Mouth; Ear; Eye; Occiput.

CHEST (including pain, intercostal neuralgia, etc. — also see: Breasts; Heart; Heart attack; Lungs; Respiratory system; etc.): Common name for the thorax, located between the diaphragm and neck. Any recurring pain or heaviness in this area — especially any discomfort that seems to radiate down the left arm — should receive prompt medical attention because it might indicate a serious heart condition.
     Organs within the chest (thorax) include: The lungs; heart; breathing/air passages; (and within the ribcage are also: The spleen; pancreas; upper portions of the

stomach and liver; diaphragm; etc.).

Pain/discomfort in the chest area may have many causes. Among the most serious of them are the following:

1. Angina (angina pectoris) — especially if it is characterized by a choking or suffocating pain (usually) in the center of the chest which also triggers a sense of fear or foreboding and which generally arises after physical exertion. Angina pains will generally cease within 15 minutes of stopping and resting;

2. Heart attack, heart failure (cardiac arrest) — especially if the pain ranges from moderate pressure to crushing or vise-like and does not respond to rest. Other common symptoms include: Grave anxiety (with a feeling death is near); shortness of breath; vomiting and retching; belching; face turning gray/ashen, especially with clammy perspiration; etc. (Note: It is probably not a heart attack — but may be angina — if pain: Is below and to the left of the nipple; stays completely on the left side; is sharp/cutting rather than a dull/squeezing sensation; comes/goes or is relieved by lying down/lasts for only several minutes);

3. Rupture of an aortic aneurysm — often mimics heart attack/heart failure;

4. Pneumothorax — especially if there is sharp pain extending from shoulder to abdomen, breathing difficulty, and follows recent disorder of in the chest area.

Other less serious/less common problems may include: Pleurisy; injury to the ribs or their muscles (especially if there is a dull, gnawing ache and/or if moving or staying in a certain position is painful); problems in the esophagus; lung disorders (e.g., abscesses, aerophagia — the swallowing of air — pneumonia, colds, etc.); indigestion; hiatal hernia; etc.

Hand points: Chest; Lungs; Heart.

CIRRHOSIS (of the liver — also see: LIVER; etc.): A destructive (atrophying) disease of the liver often associated with over-consumption of alcohol. Complete (vs. incomplete) protein is vital for regeneration.

Hand points: (?) Liver; Gallbladder; Spleen; Pancreas.

CLAVICLE (collarbone — also see: Fractures; etc.): The long bone(s) at the top of the chest stretching across to the tips of the shoulders. The following acupressure points may be helpful following fractures, etc:

Hand points: Neck; Shoulder.

COCCYX: The small, bony protrusion at the bottom of the spine, commonly called the "tailbone."

Hand points: Coccyx.

COLDS and INFLUENZA (also see accompanying symptoms such as: Cough; Headache; Nasal congestion; etc.): The word "colds" has been applied to many symptoms that come together and last for about seven days; an upper respiratory infection.

Symptoms of colds and influenza include fever, cough, dull aches and pains, nasal congestion (catarrh), etc.

Hand points: Lungs; Adrenals; C-15.

COLIC, INTESTINAL (also see: Abdomen lower, upper; Colon; Gastrointestinal system; Small intestine; etc.): Spasmodic abdominal pain, due to obstruction, twisting or cramping in the smooth muscles. In infants may be due to swallowing air, overfeeding, milk too rich, intestinal allergies, emotional distress, etc., and may be expressed by symptoms such as red face, irritability, pulling knees up to stomach or distended abdomen.

Hand points: Colon; Digestion; Liver; Stomach.

COLITIS (also see: Abdomen, lower; Gastrointestinal system, etc.): A usually chronic inflammation of the colon. Often associated with buried anger (a liver disorder) and resentment (lungs) by Oriental therapists. Some form of psychotherapy may be helpful in conjunction with the following techniques. Chronic colitis (which involves tissue changes in the colon) requires professional attention.

Hand points: Colon; Intestine, small; Liver; Digestion.

COLON (LARGE INTESTINE, including ascending, transverse, descending and sigmoid colon — also see: Abdomen, lower; Colic, intestinal; COLITIS; Constipation; Diarrhea; GASTROINTESTINAL SYSTEM; etc.): That part of the gastrointestinal tract beginning with the ileo-cecum and ending at the sigmoid flexure. Considered one of the twelve principal organs in traditional Oriental theory, it is thought to be paired with the lungs. It has a number of diverse functions. (For more in-depth techniques for healing this organ, see this author's THE NATURAL HEALER'S ACUPRESSURE HANDBOOK, VOLUME II.)

Hand points: Colon; Liver; Lungs.

CONGESTION, SINUS OR NASAL: See NASAL
CONGESTION (catarrh).

CONJUNCTIVITIS (pink eye — also see: Eye; Liver):
An inflammation and reddening of the membrane
(conjunctiva) covering the front of the eye. It is
generally considered a liver disorder by Oriental
therapists.

Hand points: Eye; Liver.

CONSTIPATION (costiveness — also see: Gastrointestinal
system): A condition wherein the bowels move infre-
quently or with great difficulty. It may be chronic or
acute and is associated with a great number of physical
or mental disturbances.
    Constipation is generally associated with liver
and/or kidney disorders by traditional Oriental therapists. There are numerous symptoms of constipation —
surprisingly, the failure to move bowels regularly is
not necessarily one of them (constipated people may
have several bowel movements daily). Included are the
following:
    1. Hemorrhoids, colitis or similar bowel disorders;
    2. Fatigue, irritability, etc.;
    3. Feeling of heaviness and/or fullness;
    4. Swollen lips (esp. lower lip);
    5. Foul breath, body odors;
    6. Gas/flatulence (chronic, not occasional);
    7. Strong-smelling urine;

8. Feeling of being "loaded";
9. Chronic feelings of grief, worry, depression, anxiety, etc.;
10. Skin eruptions, pimples, blackheads, etc.;

Hand points: Thyroid; Liver; Colon; Kidneys; Rectum.

CORNS and BUNIONS (also see: Foot; Skin; etc.): Horny layers of growth upon the skin which project inwards as well as outwards, usually caused by friction (corns); or a swelling (bursa) especially around or near the joint of the big toe upon the foot. Generally caused by ill-fitting shoes, either too pointed and/or too short and/or with heels that are too high.

Hand points: (?) Heel; Ankle.

CORONARY THROMBOSIS (myocardial infarction — also see: HEART; Heart attack, heart failure; etc.): Damage to (part of) the heart muscle from a clot of blood, most generally lodged in an artery supplying the heart. Symptoms often include: A feeling of oppression in the chest; pain beneath the sternum (breastbone), often described as squeezing, pressing or constricting; dyspnea (labored breathing) with or without pain; skin that is pale, cold and moist; etc. Any of these symptoms — especially where there is a history of heart problems — require immediate medical attention.
   The following techniques are emergency remedies only and do not replace proper medical care.

Hand points: (?) Heart; Chest.

COUGH (also see: Respiratory system; Bronchitis; Colds and influenza, etc.): This condition may arise from a number of causes and be symptomatic of many ailments. (Note: Medical attention is important for chronic coughs or bloody coughs — especially those with no apparent reason.)

Hand points: Lungs.

CRAMPS, MENSTRUAL: See MENSTRUAL DIFFICULTIES.

CRAMPS and SPASMS, MUSCULAR (also see: Leg; Pain control centers etc.): Painful, involuntary spasms of muscles anywhere in the body, but especially of the leg or foot during sleep.

Hand points: (?) Leg; Liver; Spleen.

CYSTITIS (also see: Bladder, urinary; Genitourinary system; etc.): An inflammation of the bladder. Often there is a need to urinate, but only a few drops are passed, generally accompanied by a cutting, burning sensation.

Hand points: Kidneys; Bladder (urinary); Sex organs; F-19.

DANDRUFF (seborrheic dermatitis — also see: DERMATITIS; SKIN; HAIR etc.): Falling, greasy scales of skin from the scalp, usually accompanied by itching and possibly lesions. It may affect the eyebrows as well.

Hand points: See DERMATITIS.

DEAFNESS, Sudden; Acute (also see: Ear; Hearing difficulties; etc.): Total or partial loss of hearing, often associated with inflammation or growths within the ear canal, but may stem from a number of causes. Get medical help immediately.

Hand points: Ear (inner).

DENTAL WORK (also see: Toothache; Jaw, upper; Tooth, teeth; etc.): The following acupressure points may be helpful for those who cannot have or choose not to have anesthesia for dental work. Stimulate regularly during dental work

Hand points: Mouth; Tooth, teeth; Colon.

DEPRESSION, MENTAL/EMOTIONAL (also see: FATIGUE; Hypoglycemia; etc.): Extreme sadness, melancholy or dejection which is unrealistic and not in proportion to one's actual circumstances. Often diet-related, according to traditional Oriental therapists, and has its roots in the liver, lungs and heart.

In traditional theory, depression is both a cause and effect (symptom) of disturbed blood chemistry. It is often a symptom that accompanies anemia, subclinical hypoglycemia (low blood sugar), food allergies, etc. Hypothyroidism often manifests emotionally as depression. Depression commonly follows bouts of anger (liver disorder), and is a common problem with the elderly (often because of imbalanced diet). Most prevalent in the later decades of life, depression may also be a side-effect of oral contraceptives.

Self-test: When six or more of the following symptoms are present, this indicates severe depression and generally requires professional (medical, nutritional and/or psychotherapeutic) counseling:

1. Loss of appetite (or overeating)
2. Have considered suicide often
3. Crying frequently
4. Feeling lonely often
5. Have trouble focusing mentally
6. Feeling a sense of worthlessness
7. Difficulty with memory
8. Easily upset by small matters
9. Withdrawal from family, friends, associates
10. Regular sense of fatigue
11. Little or no interest in sex
12. Sleep problems (too much or insomnia)

Hand points: Adrenals; Liver; Gallbladder.

DERMATITIS: (also see: Acne; Impetigo, eczema; Skin; etc.): An inflammation of the skin. Dry or cracked skin is often a symptom of vitamin A or B complex deficiency.

Hand points: Lungs; Colon; Thyroid.

DIABETES (diabetes mellitus — also see: Spleen; Pancreas; etc.): A complex disease resulting from the underproduction of insulin, a vital chemical in the body's handling of sugar. (Note: Acupuncture, done professionally with needles, may be very helpful in controlling diabetes).

Hand points: Liver; Spleen; Pancreas; Adrenals; Kidneys; Thyroid; Stomach; Pituitary.

DIAPHRAGM: The muscular-tendonous partition that separates the chest (thorax) from the upper abdomen.

Hand points: Chest; Stomach; Solar Plexus.

DIARRHEA (loose, runny bowels — also see: DYSENTERY; Traveler's diarrhea; Gastrointestinal system; etc.): This condition may be symptomatic of any number of minor or major problems. If the condition continues for more than several days, dehydration may occur. It is primarily a disorder of the spleen and pancreas, in traditional Oriental theory. If this condition continues, get medical attention.

Hand points: Colon; Stomach; Spleen; Liver; Gallbladder; Chest.

DIVERTICULITIS, DIVERTICULOSIS: See COLON; CONSTIPATION; GASTROINTESTINAL SYSTEM; etc.

DIZZINESS (also see: Seasickness; Travel sickness; Vertigo; etc.): An unpleasant sensation of reeling, falling and disorientation. Sudden dizziness may indicate a more severe underlying condition. Dizziness has a number of possible causes; but because the heart and/or kidneys may play an important role in this condition, if dizziness continues, seek medical attention — especially if it began suddenly.
Other common causes of dizziness include skull injuries, tumor, low blood sugar (hypoglycemia), pregnancy, poor circulation, hypertension, oral contraceptives, hyperventilation, various sedatives, and any inner ear disorder (the regulator of balance).

(Note: Dizziness arising from inner ear imbalance/ disorder is called <u>vertigo</u> — see Vertigo).

<u>Hand points</u>: <u>Head</u>; (?) Ear, inner; Eustachian tubes; Digestion; Gastrointestinal; Kidneys.

DREAMING, EXCESSIVE (also see: INSOMNIA, etc.): Frequent, sleep-disturbing mental activities which, in traditional Oriental theory, are thought to be an imbalance within the heart, small intestine, pericardium ("heart protector") and endocrine system. (Note: Dreaming may be an important indicator to the state of health — even give advance warning about impending health problems. If you suffer recurring, frequent health-related dreams, see your doctor or other health-care professional).

<u>Hand points</u>: Heart; Gallbladder.

DUODENUM: See SMALL INTESTINE.

DYSENTERY (also see: Diarrhea; Gastrointestinal system; etc.): An easily spread disease usually found in tropical, overcrowded conditions. It originates in contaminated food and/or water. There are several types of dysentery, and their symptoms include severe abdominal pain, frequent bowel movements (perhaps 25 or 30 per day — or more), loose-to-liquid stool, usually flecked with blood, pus and/or mucus. Children are most affected by this dangerous disease which is often confused with cholera. And, like cholera, <u>medical attention is urgently required</u>. (Note: Prolonged bouts of amoebic dysentery may cause other problems such as liver and/or lung abscesses, etc.).

<u>Hand points:</u> Colon; Stomach; Spleen.

DYSPEPSIA: See INDIGESTION; FLATULENCE; etc.

DYSPNEA (also see: RESPIRATORY SYSTEM; Asthma; Hysteria; etc.): Difficult or labored breathing usually symptomatic of an underlying disease or problem. It occurs when the capacity of the sufferer's breathing apparatus is temporarily unable to meet his body's demands, and often appears when breathing is reduced below 70% of maximum capacity. The sufferer may sense he is suffocating and thus panic, making the condition worse.

Since dyspnea is often a symptom of serious imbalance within the respiratory system, it is important to seek medical attention for this condition.

<u>Hand points:</u> (?) Lungs; Heart; Adrenals.

EAR (also see: Deafness, sudden, acute; HEARING DIFFICULTIES; Tinnitus; etc.): Includes the outer, middle and inner ear. A complete "micro-acupressure" healing system is found in the outer ear, making it a vital organ of health. The ear is considered to be a "product" of — and controlled by — the kidneys, according to traditional Oriental therapists. Earaches, one of the most common ear disorders, often arise from bowel problems, such as constipation.

<u>Hand points:</u> Ear; Kidneys; Bladder (urinary); Eustachian tubes.

ECZEMA: See IMPETIGO and ECZEMA.

EDEMA (dropsy): An excessive accumulation of
fluid in the body's tissues. Generally, edema is a
chronic problem. Since this condition often accompanies cardiovascular disorders, seek medical
attention.

Hand points: Kidneys; Stomach; Liver; Spleen;
Pancreas; affected bodily area.

ELBOW (including "tennis elbow" — also see: Arm;
etc.):

Hand points: Arm.

ENDOCRINE GLANDS (also see individual glands in this
system): Various glands that secrete hormones directly
into the bloodstream (vs. into another organ).
Included in this system are the thyroid, parathyroid,
thymus, pancreas, pituitary, adrenals, ovaries and
testes (testicles). In certain traditional schools of
thought (e.g., hatha yoga), this is the body's primary
system by which other organs/functions are controlled.
The glands within the system are highly interdependent,
and the substances they synthesize — hormones —
directly or indirectly control numerous bodily
functions (e.g., growth, sexual development/function,
metabolism, electrolyte balance, etc.). In short,
hormones control the rate/intensity of numerous other
biochemical or automatic functions and a dysfunction of
one gland in the system necessarily means a dysfunction
of several others. Any self-treatment of this system
should be done only with caution and restraint.

Hand points: Endocrine glands (master point); plus individual glands of the endocrine system.

EPIGLOTTIS (also see: Larynx; Throat; etc.): That elastic cartilage in the throat which protects the glottis while swallowing.

Hand points: (?) Digestion; Throat.

EPILEPSY AND EPILEPTIC SEIZURES: A brain disorder not clearly understood. There are a number of types of epileptic attacks; the most dramatic is the grand mal seizure. This may last from two to five minutes and generally includes loss of consciousness, loss of muscular control, rapid tensing and relaxing of the muscles of the extremities, etc. No pressure-point stimulation should be used during a seizure; instead, try to help the sufferer avoid injuring himself, especially his tongue. If possible, place a cloth-wrapped stick between his teeth to prevent him from biting his tongue.

The sufferer should not immediately get up and move around, as this may trigger another seizure; instead he should be made as comfortable as possible with his clothing loosened. (Note: Onset of this dysfunction usually occurs between ages three and fifteen years).

Hand points: Bladder (urinary); Intestine, small; Heart; Colon; Thyroid; Chest.

ESOPHAGUS (also see: Gastrointestinal system; Stomach; Throat; etc.): The passage extending from the pharynx to the stomach.

Hand points: (?) Digestion.

EUSTACHIAN TUBES (also see: Ear; Hearing difficulties; Neck; Throat; etc.): The auditory tube.

Hand points: Eustachian tubes.

EYES (also see: Cataracts; Conjunctivitis): According to traditional Oriental therapists, the eye is a product or "child" of the liver — disorders of the eye indicate an imbalance or malfunction in the liver (and its companion organ, the gallbladder).

Hand points: Eye; Liver; Gallbladder; Stomach; Colon.

FACE (including facial neuralgia, etc. — also see: SKIN; Head; and specific areas, such as: Ear; Eye; Mouth; etc.):

Hand points: All fingers plus pads and webbing at base of fingers on the palms.

FATIGUE: Tiredness and lack of energy due to physical and/or mental exertion. Generally less serious than exhaustion, it is a substantial, though temporary, loss of strength.
    "Low energy" is one of the most common complaints from a person suffering from hypoglycemia, anemia, depression, "hidden" food allergies, etc. Since each of these may be a medical condition, if fatigue continues, seek professional attention.

<u>Hand points:</u> Endocrine glands (do not overstimulate).

FEAR CONTROL CENTERS: (also see: Hysteria; etc.):
A physical and/or mental reaction to a real or imagined
situation. In traditional Oriental thought, fear
"belongs" to the kidneys and urinary bladder.

<u>Hand points:</u> Endocrine glands (do not overstimulate);
Kidneys;

FERTILITY (to promote fertility in females and males
— also see: Birth control; Genitourinary system;
Sexual drive; etc.): The difficulty or inability to
conceive may be physical and/or emotional, and is often
diet-related or diet-correctable.

In an otherwise healthy male or female, there may
be environmental factors affecting the ability to
conceive (e.g., male sterility may be related to a
chemical used in polyurethane mattresses, etc.).

<u>Hand points:</u> (?) Sex organs; Kidneys; Ovary;
Testicles.

FEVER CONTROL CENTERS: Fever is that state of
bodily temperature beyond the normal 98.6° F. or
37° C. It is a defense mechanism; the body produces
an inhospitable climate for "intruders," foreign bodies, parasites, etc., in an effort to remove their
threat to the system. It is a natural process and may
be symptomatic of many problems. (Note: Fever is a
beneficial defensive and cleansing reaction — it is
probably best to avoid trying to interfere with this
vital process unless the fever is dangerously high).

<u>Hand points</u>: Hypothalamus; Pituitary.

FINGERS: See hand.

FITS: See EPILEPSY and EPILEPTIC SEIZURES; etc.

FLATULENCE (also see: Abdomen, lower; Indigestion; Gastrointestinal system; etc.): The presence of excessive gas in the stomach, intestine or anywhere in the gastrointestinal system. (Note: Flatulence arises from liver/gallbladder activity, in traditional Oriental theory. It is "normal" — that is, when consuming the average, Western diet — to expel gas ten to fifteen times daily; substantially more than that probably indicates at least a "hidden" food allergy and/or repressed, hostile emotions).

<u>Hand points</u>: Liver; Colon; Gallbladder.

FLU: See COLDS and INFLUENZA.

FOOT (including ankle, toes, etc.):

<u>Hand points</u>: Heel; Ankle; <u>Forehead</u> (esp. toe pains).

FOREHEAD (also see: Face; Head; etc.):

Hand points: Forehead; Head.

FRACTURES (broken bone — also see Bones; specific area where the fracture has occurred such as Arm, etc.): A broken or splintered bone. Acupressure techniques do not replace standard Western first-aid or emergency measures such as splints, casts, or other immobilizing wrappings and coverings.

Hand points: Use corresponding affected area.

FRIGIDITY (sexual — also see SEXUAL DRIVE; Sexual organs, etc.): Sexual unresponsiveness within a female partner. (Note: A much more in-depth program for healing sexual disorders is found in this author's book, HOW TO ENJOY SEX MORE WITH ACUGENICS).

Hand points: Hypothalamus; Kidneys; Lungs; Heart; Spleen.

FROSTBITE (including: Chilblain; Immersion Foot; Pernio; and Trench Foot — also see: Skin; and specific areas affected, etc.): The result of prolonged exposure to damp or dry cold. The most severe condition is frostbite, where the tissue of the affected part of the body is destroyed by freezing. Blood circulation is stopped to the affected area; unless rapidly treated, this will become gangrenous and amputation may be required.

Currently there is general agreement among authorities that immediate thawing in warm water as soon as the threat of refreezing passes is the best choice. But it will be painful. Never rub a frost-bitten area, even with snow. Get medical help immediately.

-48-

<u>Hand points</u>: Lungs; plus corresponding bodily area points.

GALLBLADDER (also see: Flatulence; Liver; Indigestion; etc.): A hollow organ located near the liver, in the upper right-hand quarter of the abdomen area, beneath or behind the ribcage. Its function is the accumulation and storage of mucus and bile. Pain or discomfort in that part of the upper abdomen, especially after eating, could indicate gallbladder or liver problems.

In traditional Oriental theory, the gallbladder is one of the primary twelve organs and is mated with the liver, the organ from which it "blooms" during fetal development. As such, its emotional "chores" are <u>anger</u>, decision-making, <u>depression</u>, etc. Symptoms of disorder and imbalance within this organ include: Flatulence; pain or colic in the upper, right quadrant of the abdomen; nausea; bowel distress; difficulty in making decisions for oneself; and, of course, Gallstones. (Note: About half of all gallbladder "attacks" occur from April through May; in traditional Oriental theory, this corresponds to, the time — spring — when the gallbladder and liver organ "team" are most active. For more in-depth techniques for healing this organ, see this author's THE NATURAL HEALER'S ACUPRESSURE HANDBOOK, VOLUME II.)

<u>Hand points</u>: Liver; Gallbladder.

GALLSTONES (also see: GALLBLADDER): Crystallized bits of bile, composed primarily of cholesterol. This condition — which afflicts females far more often than males — is so common (esp. in older people) that as many as one person in five suffers from gallstones by age 65. (Note: Cancer of the gallbladder is nearly always preceded by gallstones.) The period of pregnancy is also a typical time for gallstones to form. While the existence of gallstones may be symptom-free until they actually pass, common symptoms include cramping pain (which has been compared to childbirth), bloating, belching, food intolerance, bad breath, etc. Gallstones may mimic brain tumors, appendicitis, pancreatitis, ulcers, etc.

Hand points: Liver; Gallbladder; Pancreas.

GASTRITIS (acid indigestion — also see: STOMACH; Flatulence; Gastrointestinal system; Indigestion; etc.): Inflammation of the stomach, usually due to acid/alkaline imbalance. Symptoms of too much or too little stomach acid (HCL) may be similar.

Hand points: Stomach; Liver; Spleen; Pancreas; Gastrointestinal.

GASTROINTESTINAL SYSTEM (also see: Abdomen, lower and upper; Flatulence; Indigestion; Stomach; etc.): The stomach and intestinal portions of the digestive tract.

Hand points: Stomach; Liver; Gallbladder; Intestine, small; Colon; Spleen; Pancreas; B8 (esp. spasm); D15; GASTROINTESTINAL.

GENITAL WEAKNESS, PAIN and/or DYSFUNCTION: See GONORRHEA; SEXUAL ORGANS; etc.

GENITOURINARY SYSTEM (also see: Kidneys; Bladder, urinary; Cystitis; Urinary control centers; SEXUAL DRIVE; Sexual organs; etc.): The system whose job is the excretion of urine; it includes the kidneys, urinary bladder, ureters and urethra, as well as the internal and external organs of reproduction (sex organs). (Note: In good health, urine should be slightly acidic — with a pH of about 5.5 — especially upon the morning's first urination.)

Hand points: Kidneys; Bladder (urinary); Urethra; Sex organs; Adrenals; F-18, 19 (esp. nocturia — frequent urination at night).

GINGIVITIS (bleeding gums, unhealthy gums — also see: MOUTH; TOOTH, TEETH; Toothache; etc.): A condition which may be disease-linked, although more often arises from improper and irregular care of the gums and teeth.

Hand points: (?) Colon (all); Lungs; Mouth; Tooth, teeth.

GLANDS, SWOLLEN: See LYMPH GLANDS.

GLAUCOMA (also see: EYE; etc.): A group of disorders of the eye, characterized by abnormal elevation of intraocular pressure, hardening of the eyeball, restricted field of vision, halos seen around artificial lights and a general loss of visual power.
    If glaucoma is suspected — or there is a family history of this disorder — get a complete physical eye examination (not just a tonometric pressure reading, since this can be misleading).

Hand points: Eye; (?) Liver.

GONORRHEA (also see: Sexual organs; etc.): A venereal disease primarily involving the mucous membranes of the genitourinary tract and/or rectum. Sometimes the eye is involved, as well. Its symptoms include painful urination, pus seepage from the urinary tract, and various genitourinary infections Gonorrhea is primarily spread by sexual intercourse. Get medical help immediately both for treatment and to help stop the spread of this disease.

Hand points: (?) Sex organs.

GOUT (also see: Arthritis): A recurrent attack of acute arthritis that mostly strikes the big toe. The main symptom is mild-to-excruciating pain in or about the big toe. Sometimes crystal formations are found along the edges of the ear. Gout is caused by the improper metabolism of uric acid and may be triggered by an excess of wine or various rich foods.

Hand points: Affected bodily area.

HAIR (esp. graying — also see: Baldness; Dandruff; etc.): Hair (on the head) is thought to be a product of — and thus controlled by — the kidneys (and/or lungs), by traditional Oriental therapists. As such, it is part of the excretory system.

Hand points: Thyroid (use cautiously).

HAND (including fingers — also see: Arm; Wrist; etc):

Hand points: (?) Wrist.

HANGOVER (also see: Flatulence; Indigestion; Intoxication; etc.): The disagreeable aftereffects from drug or alcohol abuse. Its symptoms often include nausea, headache, indigestion, diarrhea, etc. If this condition occurs after taking only a small amount of the intoxicant, it generally indicates an allergy to the intoxicant or one of its ingredients.

Hand points: (?) Stomach; Liver.

HAY FEVER (also see: Allergies, non-specific; Eyes; Nasal congestion; etc.): Common name for allergic rhinitis. Hay fever is a catchall term to describe a loosely knit group of allergic reactions triggered by pollination of various plants or weeds.

Hand points: Nose; Sinuses; Lungs.

HEAD (also see: Ear; Eyes; Face; Headache; Mouth; Neck; Whiplash; etc.): Any injury to the head is potentially dangerous. Signs of shock should be carefully watched for as well as signs of concussion. Fracture of the skull should be suspected, especially if there are differences between the size of the pupils, or bleeding from the nose, ears and/or mouth. Keep the victim quiet and get medical help immediately.

Hand points: Brain; Pineal; Pituitary; Forehead; Head.

HEADACHES (also see: Head; Migraine; Pain control centers etc.): May be symptomatic of many problems and diseases. If headache persists, or is a frequent problem, get medical help. The following headaches which require prompt professional attention are those that: Strike without apparent cause; awaken you from a deep sleep; are accompanied by confusion or convulsions; change character after having a long history of sameness; are constant, daily or frequent; are localized in a specific place (e.g., in ear, eye, etc.); follow a blow to the head; are recurrent in children.

"Common" headaches (there are more than 60 kinds of headache) are usually a symptom of imbalance within the digestive organs, and are frequently triggered by stress and tension.

Hand points: Liver; Spleen; Stomach; Gallbladder; Colon (all); Adrenals; Head.

HEARING DIFFICULTIES (also see: Deafness; Ear; etc.): Hearing is associated with the kidneys, in traditional Oriental theory. There are three major kinds of hearing loss: Nerve loss (aging, following fever, etc.); con-ductive loss (build-up of earwax, etc.); funct-ional loss (often psychological). Hearing difficulties may also forewarn of heart and/or kidney disorders (esp. inner ear disorders).

Hand points: Ear; Kidneys; Bladder (urinary) Eustachian tubes.

HEART (also see: Angina pectoris; Chest; Heart attack, heart failure; etc.): One of the twelve primary organs in traditional Oriental theory, the heart — and its companion organ, the small intestine — are primarily responsible for blood (and energy) circulation. It is considered the "king" of organs and the most vulnerable — thus, except when no alternatives exist, self-treatment of any known heart conditions should be avoided.

Early warning signs of potential heart failure include: Edema; (esp. of the ankles); breathlessness following mild exercise (e.g., after climbing stairs); a hacking-type cough that immediately ceases when one stands up but comes on when lying down or sitting); enlarged fingertips and/or nose; frequent urination at night; tiny lumps, nodules or blood spots under skin; raised orange spots under the skin, especially around the wrist; double-jointed wrists and fingers, accompanied by skin and hands that bruise easily; long, thin spider-like fingers that seem to be double- jointed; aggressive, time-urgent and competitive behavior, among others. (Note: Unusual depression and/or fatigue — as well as a reduced sexual drive and numerous other "unrelated" symptoms — may also be early warning indicators of heart disease, attack, etc. (For more in-depth techniques for healing this organ, see this author's THE NATURAL HEALER'S ACUPRESSURE HANDBOOK, VOLUME II.)

Hand points: Heart; Intestine, small; Bladder (urinary); E-18 (palpitations); the entire pad below the base of the thumb, in the palm of the left hand (C-15, 16).

HEART ATTACK, HEART FAILURE (also see: Angina pectoris; Chest; Coronary thrombosis; Heart; Pain control centers Tachycardia paroxysmal; etc.): A major disturbance of the heart caused by either blockage of a coronary artery (heart attack) or inadequate pumping of the heart (heart failure). Symptoms of heart attack include severe pain or crushing pressure beneath the breastbone (sternum), a feeling of apprehension, shortness of breath, profuse sweating, and nausea and/or vomiting. The pain may first appear on the left side of the upper body before moving into the chest.

Symptoms of heart failure include edema (swelling of hands and feet), bluish-purple coloring of the skin, lips, fingernails, ears, etc., chest pains, anxiety and shortness of breath, especially when lying down. Get medical help immediately, and do not consume food or water when any heart disturbance is suspected.

Emergency tactics: A) If heart attack occurs, force yourself to cough constantly until you can reach help; since there are only about 10-20 seconds before losing consciousness, begin coughing immediately (forced coughing simulates cardiopulmonary resuscitation or CPR) and/or B) Bite the tips of fifth (little) fingers (inside and outside, not top and bottom — this triggers two vital acupressure points).

Hand points: (?) Heart; also deeply and continuously knead C-15, 16 (left hand only).

HEATSTROKE: A potentially fatal, heat-exposure syndrome — often associated with underlying health problems — which is characterized by HOT, DRY SKIN; high fever; red skin; prostration; possibly unconsciousness and shock; etc. These occur from loss of bodily fluids, especially from slowed or ceased perspiration. There are several crucial steps to be taken:
   1. Call for medical help immediately;
   2. Take steps to get fever down — cover/immerse victim in cool water or sponge with alcohol or use fever control acupressure points or feed up to 10 grains of aspirin (after moving victim into a cool — at least shaded — location and loosening tight clothing). Note: Do not bring victim's temperature below 101° F.; take temperature every ten minutes;

3. Restore bodily fluids (and stimulate perspiration-production "mechanism") — Give a hot (pref.) or cool (but not cold or icy) liquid, preferably adding a 1/2 tsp. of salt per glass (feed half a glass each 15 minutes, allowing small sips only);
4. Keep head and shoulders slightly raised;
5. Repeat process as necessary.

Hand points: A-18; F-20; C-21; D-22, E-22, F-22.

HEEL (also see: Foot; etc.): Chronic heel problems may be an early warning indicator of heart problems.

Hand points: Heel.

HEMORRHAGE (bleeding — also see: Menstrual difficulties; Nosebleed; and specific affected body areas): Blood flows through vessels such as veins and arteries, carrying oxygen and food to the cells and carrying away waste. If something happens to rupture the vessels, blood escapes; or disease may allow the blood to escape through unruptured vessels (diapedisis). Both are considered as hemorrhage; if enough blood escapes, death occurs. Arterial bleeding must be stopped immediately.

Hand points: Corresponding bodily area; E-18 (esp. menorrhagia — vaginal bleeding between periods).

HEMORRHOIDS (piles — also see: Anus; Pain control centers Rectum; etc.): An enlarged, expanded vein in the lower rectal and/or anal wall. Complications may include inflammation, bleeding, pain and/or itching and possibly clotting (thrombosis). Permanently curing hemorrhoids usually means a change in diet, toilet habits and/or mental attitudes.

Hemorrhoids — which are common during pregnancy — are caused by excess pressure on the rectum (usually from constipation or unassimilated foods). They are often accompanied by gum problems and disorders. Hemorrhoids which bleed are common, but regular bleeding from the anus requires medical attention.

Hand points: Anus; Colon (all); Rectum; Perineum; Spleen.

HEPATITIS: See LIVER. This is an inflammation of the liver which is dangerous and may be communicable. Get medical help immediately. (Note: If skin has yellow pallor or cast, see JAUNDICE).

Hand points: (?) Liver; Bladder (urinary); Gallbladder.

HERNIA (rupture — also see: Abdomen, lower etc.): An abnormal protrusion of the intestine through the abdominal muscle wall or cavity. Hernia is often caused by lifting an excessive weight or improperly hoisting a load. Ordinarily, a small-to-large bulge will appear somewhere upon the abdomen; and there may be some pain. The ultimate danger lies in the possibility of cutting off the source of blood to the protruding bowel.

Hand points: Corresponding bodily points.

HERPES SIMPLEX VIRUS II (genital herpes — also see Shingles; etc.): A highly contagious viral infection primarily of the genital and/or anal areas. (Note: Techniques should be started at the first hint of an impending outbreak.)

Hand points: (?) Affected bodily points.

HERPES ZOSTER VIRUS: See SHINGLES.

HIGH BLOOD PRESSURE: See HYPERTENSION.

HIP (also see: Buttocks; etc.):

Hand points: Hip.

HIVES AND RASH (urticaria — also see: Allergies, non-specific; Skin; etc.): Sudden or rapid appearance of intensive, itching welts on the skin. They may appear in crops over wide areas of the body, tend to last a day or so, and are generally associated with allergic reactions.

In severe cases, hives may affect the mucous membrane areas; edema may constrict the vocal area (glottis), creating possibly fatal distress. Get medical help immediately.

Hand points: Use corresponding bodily area points.

HOARSENESS (also see: Laryngitis; Throat; etc.): Irritated or phlegm-coated throat and vocal area, causing raspy or strained voice. Chronic hoarseness should have medical attention.

Hand points: (?) Lungs; Chest; Throat; Tonsils.

HUNGER CONTROL CENTERS: To temporarily ease
or stop hunger. For further information and
techniques, see this author's "HOW TO LOSE
WEIGHT EASILY WITH ACUGENICS."

Hand points: (?) Digestion; Stomach; Liver; Gallbladder.

HYPERACTIVITY: A state of restlessness and frequent
movement, especially found in children.

Hand points: See HYPOGLYCEMIA, NERVOUSNESS, etc.

HYPERTENSION (high blood pressure): Its symptoms are
as vague as the origin of the disease. Besides
increased blood pressure, there may be dizziness,
fatigue, insomnia, palpitations, weakness and
headaches, etc. Hypertension occurs from the
constricture of blood vessels, caused either by fats
(and other "mechanical" processes) or through fear or
other psychophysical means, but the result is similar
— blood is forced through too small an opening. For
the most part, hypertension appears to be a defense
mechanism that has gotten "stuck."
     Untreated hypertension is dangerous — take steps
immediately and get professional advice. Nearly
always, high blood pressure is at least partially
food-related — important changes in diet are essential; and if taken, such steps are often enough to
control hypertension without drugs or medications (see
this author's A WAY OF EATING FOR PLEASURE
AND HEALTH).

Hand points: (?) Kidneys; Adrenals; Colon (all).

HYPOGLYCEMIA (low blood sugar — also see: Diabetes
mellitus; Spleen; Pancreas; FATIGUE; etc.): A condition
about which little is known, but is thought by some
nutrition authorities to affect millions. The problem
is too much insulin and/or not enough "blood sugar,"
which may trigger insulin shock in severe cases. Its
symptoms may be similar to diabetes mellitus, a problem
with which it is often confused.

While "hypoglycemia" means "low blood sugar," in its
pre-clinical, common form, it is coming to mean an
umbrella-syndrome that includes numerous symptoms
(e.g., anger, fatigue, etc.) that are primarily
triggered by an allergy to sugar or sugary foods and
drinks.

Hpoglycemia typically occurs about two/three hours
following a meal (sooner — usually within a half-hour
— following sugary foods, smoking, taking alcoholic
and/or caffeinated drinks, etc.). Its symptoms include:
Flushing; pallid/sallow skin; feeling of faintness;
hyperactivity (esp. in children); IRRITABILITY; low
emotional control; chills; HUNGER; trembling;
headaches; dizziness; weakness; convulsions; etc.

Hand points: (?) Liver; Spleen; Pancreas; Adrenals;
Heart; Kidneys; Bladder (urinary); Gallbladder;
Intestine, small; Pituitary; Brain.

HYSTERIA (also see: Fear control centers; etc.):
Panicky, severe fear whose symptoms may include
sweating, palpitations, tension and fatigue,
irrationality, undefined terror and sense of impending
calamity, etc. Urinary or bowel urgency may occur.
While hysteria is common with prepubescent and
pubescent children, it may indicate problems of a
severe nature in adults. Get medical help
immediately.

<u>Hand points:</u> Digestion; <u>B-16</u>.

ILEO-CECUM (also see: Colon; <u>Gastrointestinal system</u>;
Small intestine; etc.): The "doorway" between the small
intestine and the colon, found in the lower right
quadrant of the abdomen. In Oriental literature, it is
said to be "controlled" by the kidneys.

<u>Hand points:</u> Ileo-cecum.

IMPETIGO and ECZEMA (also see: Skin, etc.): Skin
disorders whose symptoms are crusty, yellowish
formations and pustules (impetigo) or drier, more
reddened lesions (eczema); or they may look similar.

<u>Hand points:</u> (?) Adrenals; Kidneys; Lungs; plus
corresponding body area points.

IMPOTENCE (Sexual — also see: SEXUAL DRIVE; Sexual
organs; etc.): Inability in a male to have complete
sexual intercourse. It is common for most males to
suffer this condition occasionally. But when this
condition (primarily an affliction of the kidneys, in
traditional Oriental theory) occurs more than 25% of
the time, it probably indicates severe, nutritional
imbalance — often alcoholism (or may be a side-effect
of present medication, drug abuse, etc.). At that
point, professional help is suggested, especially since
frequent impotence may also be a symptom of an
underlying organic disorder (e.g., diabetes).
    The healthy male should be able to have a satisfying
sex life for his entire life. Impotence generally
results from insufficient blood to the penis, malfunctioning nervous system or abnormal amounts of male
hormones.

In a healthy male, sexual desire is strongest in cool or cold weather and is lowest in hot weather, when frequent sexual orgasms tend to damage the kidneys and heart.

More complete information on this subject is found in this author's HOW TO ENJOY SEX MORE WITH ACUGENICS.

Hand points: Liver; Spleen; Pancreas; Heart; Kidneys; Bladder (urinary); Sex organs; Prostate.

INDIGESTION (also see: Flatulence; Gastritis; Gastrointestinal system; Stomach; etc.): A temporary disorder of the digestive tract often caused by overeating, alcohol abuse or nervousness, etc. Its symptoms include flatulence and discomfort in the upper or lower abdomen, etc.

Hand points: Gastrointestinal (also see: GASTROINTESTINAL SYSTEM).

INFECTION: The "invasion" of the body by various organisms such as hostile bacteria or viruses.

Hand points: Use corresponding bodily area points.

INFLAMMATIONS (also see: Arthritis; Sores; affected bodily areas; etc.): The reaction of tissue to injury, etc., characterized by soreness, heat, swelling, etc.

Hand points: Use corresponding bodily area points.

INFLUENZA: See COLDS and INFLUENZA.

INSOMNIA: Sleeplessness and mild restlessness; prolonged difficulty in getting to sleep.
Hand points: Liver; Gallbladder; Kidneys; Bladder (urinary); Spleen; Pancreas.

INTESTINAL PROBLEMS: See CONSTIPATION; DIARRHEA; DYSENTERY; GASTROINTESTINAL SYSTEM; FLATULENCE; INDIGESTION; PAIN; etc.

INTOXICATION (also see: Hangover; Indigestion; etc.): Mild or severe poisioning from the abuse of alcohol, medication, or drugs. (Note: The following acupressure techniques are for emergency use only — intoxication is one of the contraindicated conditions for acupressure).
Hand points: (?) Liver; Spleen; Lungs; Pancreas.

ITCHING; ITCHY SKIN (also see: SKIN; Impetigo and eczema; etc.): Frequent itching may be an early warning of kidney disorder, diabetes mellitus, gout, thyroid dysfunction or even leukemia, cancer (carcinoma) or Hodgkin's Disease. If itching continues or increases, seek medical attention and diagnosis. (Note: Itchy skin — esp. if repeatedly in a specific area — may be the system's "shout" for acupuncture upon that point; itching at various acupoints about the skin is the body-mind's own way of doing acupuncture therapy upon itself.)

Hand points: (?) Liver; Bladder (urinary); Gallbladder; Spleen; Stomach; Colon (all).

-64-

JAUNDICE (also see: Liver; etc.): Yellowing of the skin or mucous membranes, and secretions with bile pigment. Jaundice may occur from a number of causes, but is generally disease-linked. The liver is primarily or secondarily affected; this is the bile-producing organ. Jaundice that appears suddenly — or suddenly deepens — may indicate passage and lodging of a gallstone in the common bile duct, causing the bile to become blocked, thus yellowing the skin. (Note: Jaundice is very common in newborn infants — some doctors feel that an allergy to breast milk may be involved.)

Hand points: (?) Adrenals; Kidneys; Liver; Lungs.

JAW, LOWER (also see: Dental work; Jaw, upper; Mouth; Toothache; etc.): Jaw pain, difficulty in chewing, may indicate vitamin B complex deficiency.

Hand points: Mouth; Tooth, teeth.

JAW, UPPER (also see: Dental work; Jaw, lower; Mouth; Toothache; etc.):

Hand points: Mouth; Tooth, teeth.

KIDNEYS (also see: Back, lower and/or upper; Bladder, urinary; GENITOURINARY SYSTEM; KIDNEY STONES; NEPHRITIS; etc.): The pair of primary organs, located in the body at the level of the elbows, which are the "parents" of the genitourinary system. In traditional Oriental theory, the kidneys — and their companion organ, the urinary bladder — are responsible for "producing" the responses to fear, sexual hunger, etc. They are also said to control hearing and hair (on the head). (For more in-depth techniques for healing this organ, see this author's THE NATURAL HEALER'S ACUPRESSURE HANDBOOK, VOLUME II).

Hand points: Kidneys; Adrenals; Bladder (urinary).

KIDNEY STONES: See GENITOURINARY SYSTEM; KIDNEYS; STONES, KIDNEY OR BLADDER, etc.

KNEE (also see: Foot; Leg; Thigh; etc.): Hand points: Leg; Forehead.

LARYNGITIS (also see: Bronchitis; Colds and influenza; Hoarseness; Larynx; Respiratory systems; Throat; etc.): An inflammation of the larynx or voice box which causes a hoarseness or inability to vocalize sound. Chronic or acute, it may be caused by a number of factors.

Hand points: Lungs; Throat.

LARYNX (also see: Laryngitis; Pharnyx; RESPIRATORY SYSTEM; Throat; etc.): The "voice box," found between the tongue and the trachea. It is part of the respiratory system and is controlled by the lungs.

Hand points: Lungs; Throat.

LEG (also see: Foot; Knee; Thigh: etc. — for leg cramps, see CRAMPS SPASMS MUSCULAR):

Hand points: Leg; Waist.

LEG CRAMPS (at night): See CRAMPS and SPASMS.

LIVER (also see: Gallbladder; Indigestion; Jaundice; Spleen; Pancreas; etc.): The largest gland or secreting organ in the body. Its functions are not totally understood, but it plays a major role in the digestive process. Symptoms of a liver disorder may include pain and/or discomfort behind the bottom of the rib cage and are sometimes confused with problems of the gallbladder.

In traditional Oriental theory, the liver produces — or is "responsible" for — the eyes, muscles, moving the bowels, flatulence, aggressive drive, anger, depression, etc. It is a primary organ for vitality and physical force or strength. The liver — and its companion, the gallbladder — also produce digestive enzymes and act as a filter between the heart and intestine, producing red blood cells and processing waste nitrogen into urea. The liver is the body's fastest "self-regenerator" organ. (For more in-depth techniques for healing this organ, see this author's THE NATURAL HEALER'S ACUPRESSURE HANDBOOK, VOLUME II.)

Hand points: Liver; Gallbladder; Spleen; Pancreas; Bladder (urinary).

LOW BLOOD SUGAR: See HYPOGLYCEMIA.

LUMBAGO (also see: Back, lower and/or upper; Pain control centers Sciatica; etc.): Aching in the lower to middle back region.

Hand points: See BACK.

LUNGS (also see: Asthma; Bronchitis; Colon; Cough; Chest; Respiratory system; etc.): Primary organs for handling air and which, in traditional Oriental theory, are coupled with the colon (large intestine). They "control" the nose and breathing passages, the sense of smell, the skin (and bodily — not scalp — hair); the emotions they produce/store are thought to be, in part, grief, anxiety, resentment and sorrow. The lungs play a critical part in the regulation of bodily temperature (via perspiration) and the elimination of fluids from the body. They are also the "home" of animal drive, sense of reason and wisdom, the sense of survival and the will to live. (For more in-depth techniques for healing this organ, see this author's THE NATURAL HEALER'S ACUPRESSURE HANDBOOK, VOLUME II.)

Hand points: Chest; Lungs.

LYMPH GLANDS or NODES (also see: SPLEEN; etc.): The system for carrying lymph (a bodily fluid) that involves the following glands: Pineal; pituitary; adrenals; thymus; thyroid; tonsils; appendix; adenoids; and various other nodes. Its primary chore is cleansing blood of impurities. In traditional Oriental theory, the "Triple Warmer" (a body-regulation function that has no Western counterpart) is said to control the lymph system, while the spleen (including the pancreas) and its companion organ, the stomach, are said to be the "parents" of this system. (NOTE: All following acupressure points to be used with restraint and caution.)

Hand points: Adrenals; Appendix; Mastoid; Pancreas; Pineal; Pituitary; Spleen; Stomach; Thyroid; Tonsils; Thymus.

MASTITIS (also see: BREASTS; etc.): An inflammation of the breast, in which the breast becomes swollen, reddened, knotty and/or tender to the touch. It is frequent among nursing mothers.

Hand points: (?) Chest; Stomach.

MASTOID PROCESS: (also see: Ear; etc.): The breast or nipple-shaped bone of the skull, just behind the ear.

Hand points: Mastoid.

MENOPAUSE (also see: MENSTRUAL DIFFICULTIES; etc.): The so-called "change of life" experienced by females in middle age, considered to have occurred when a female stops her period for over a year. Those who begin menstruation early are characteristically the last to undergo menopause.

The most noticeable symptom is a gradual-to-sudden cessation of menstruation. Other symptoms of this condition may include "hot flashes," itching skin, constipation, heart palpitations, headache, dizziness, emotional changes, etc. (Note: Males also undergo menopause, which is chiefly characterized by shrinkage of sex organs and the emotional discomfort which that may bring.) Discontinuance of the production of hormones (estrogen and progesterone) and menopause are linked intimately together. Endocrine changes in younger women can cause hormonal disruption, bringing on early menopause. (Note: Menopause is not an absolute time clock process, though it is extremely common — there are reports of 70-and-80 year-old females giving birth to healthy babies. Acupressure techniques may delay/ease the onset/difficulty of menopause, being especially helpful in the continued production of female hormones.)

<u>Hand points:</u> (?) Uterus; Pituitary; Brain.

MENSTRUAL DIFFICULTIES: (including Dysmenorrhea, Menorrhagia, Leukorrhea, etc. — also see: Ovaries; Abdomen, lower; Pain control centers Sexual organs; etc.): Female reproductive organs generally function well for about 30 years after onset of menstruation (monthly fertility cycle). Slight variations in cycle or accompanying symptoms are not significant; but sudden and/or major changes — such as complete cessation of menstruation even when not pregnant — require immediate medical attention (esp. non-menstrual vaginal bleeding).

Menstrual difficulties may include: Menorrhagia (loss of large amounts of blood); dysmenorrhea (painful menstruation); amenorrhea (absence of menstrual period); leukorrhea or the "the whites" (non-bloody vaginal discharge); etc.

<u>Hand points:</u> Thyroid; Spleen; Stomach; Kidneys; Bladder (urinary); Liver; E-18 (esp. dysmenorrhea).

MIGRAINE (also see: Headache; etc.): A particularly severe headache, often said to be associated with a malfunctioning liver by Oriental doctor-philosophers. It is characterized by periodic, rapid onsets that often center in or around one or both eyes and may be accompanied by other painful, unpleasant symptoms. Vomiting, nausea, loss of appetite and strength are not uncommon.

True migraine — often called "sick headache" — differs from the many other kinds of headaches (some doctors claim there are more than 60 types of headaches) in that it usually occurs on <u>one side of the head</u> and follows a rather <u>consistent pattern.</u> <u>Disturbance in vision</u> is also a common symptom for this tension-related headache.

The "migraine personality" is one that is tense, rigid, hard-driving, conscientious and always striving for perfection. Psychotherapy — with the goal of loosening, easing and relaxing these personality aspects — may be most helpful.

Nearly 75% of all migraines are suffered by females, especially near their menstrual periods. Migraine is often hereditary and is thought to affect about 5% of the population.

Hand points: (?) Liver; Lungs.

MOUTH (also see: Dental work; Face; Gingivitis; Head; Jaw, lower; Jaw, upper; Palate, Parotid gland; Tongue; Toothache; etc.): The mouth is one of the body's most vulnerable areas to disturbances in nutrition, the endocrine system and in the process of metabolism. Common symptoms of mouth disorders include: Canker sores; cold sores (herpes facialis); thrush (mouth ulcers); cracking at corners of mouth (cheilosis); chapped lips; foul and sticky mouth and tongue (usually indicates a liver imbalance); etc.

Hand points: Mouth; Parotid; Stomach; Spleen; Pancreas; Liver; D-18 (oral ulcer).

MULTIPLE SCLEROSIS (also see: Nerves; etc.): A disease of the central nervous system that primarily affects the white matter of the brain and spinal cord. It is a progressively degenerative disorder that tends to occur in "bouts" (some of which are triggered by high fever, injuries, pregnancy, etc.). Some of its many symptoms include blurred/double vision; speech difficulties; weakness in limbs; loss of bladder/bowel control; loss of balance; difficulty in walking; etc.

The disease tends to recur frequently with decreasing spans of "relief time" between bouts. While depression occurs, many M.S. patients exude a surprising sense of cheerfulness and optimism.

Hand points: Brain; Spinal cord; Kidneys; Stomach; Spleen; Pancreas; Liver; Gallbladder.

MUMPS: An acute, painful and contagious viral disease. Its symptoms are generally an enlargement of one or both salivary glands — especially the parotid gland (located in front of and below the ear) — but may include attacks on other tissues such as the testicles, pancreas, etc.

Mumps is more dangerous to adults — especially adult males — than to children. It occurs mostly in the winter and spring months. Usually, a case of childhood mumps gives lifelong protection, and nearly a third of the people who contract this disease never realize they've had it.

Symptoms of mumps include pain under the ear (preceded by chills, fever, loss of appetite and/or headache, etc.); swelling of the parotid gland; puffiness on (usually only) one side of the face; difficulty in swallowing; etc. This usually lasts for a week to 10 days.

Hand points: (?) Adrenals; Mouth; Neck; Parotid; Testicles; Throat.

MUSCLES (also see: Cramps and spasms, muscular; Sprains, muscular; Strains, muscular; etc.): Muscles are sub-organs of the body which, in traditional Oriental theory, are "children" of the liver and gallbladder; to a certain extent, they are also controlled by the spleen, pancreas and stomach.

Hand points: See specific areas; Muscles; Liver; Gallbladder; Spleen; Pancreas; Stomach.

NASAL CONGESTION (catarrh — also see: Colds and influenza; Hayfever; Nose; Sinusitis; etc.): An inflammation of the nasal passages' mucous membranes combined with a mucus discharge.

Hand points: Lungs; Nose; Sinuses; Colon (all); Stomach.

NECK (also see: Whiplash; etc.):

Hand points: Neck.

NEPHRITIS (acute — also see: Genitourinary system; Kidneys, etc.): Inflammation of the kidneys. When chronic, it is called "Bright's Disease." It is usually characterized by: Fatigue; reduced sexual drive; lowered vitality; albumin in the urine; swelling in various parts of the body; etc. Nausea, vomiting and enlargement of the abdomen are also common.

Hand points: Kidneys; Adrenals.

NERVES (nervous system — also see Brain; NERVOUS-NESS; etc.): The control system for all muscular movements, including the brain, central and peripheral nervous system and spinal cord. Primary damage to the nervous system arises usually from poor nutrition and/or dysfunction of the endocrine glands.

Diseases of the nervous system include — but are not limited to — Parkinson's disease; multiple sclerosis; myasthenia gravis; neuralgia; neuritis; epilepsy; muscular dystrophy; Tay-Sach's disease; rheumatoid arthritis; etc.

Hand points: Brain; Nerves: Stomach; Kidneys; Bladder (urinary); Adrenals.

NERVOUSNESS (also see: Anxiety; Fear control centers; etc.): A state of mental and/or physical disarray, characterized by a lack of mental poise and composure, restlessness, impulsive and/or irrational behavior, purposeless activity, etc.

Nervousness is a catchall word that often refers to symptoms that have little to do with the nervous system, but are actually low-level fear reactions (kidney-urinary bladder imbalance).

Hand points: (?) Stomach; Kidneys; Endocrine glands; Bladder (urinary).

NEURALGIA (also see: Pain control centers specific areas affected, such as Arm; Hand; Trigeminal Neuralgia, etc.): Aching sensitivity or brief, stabbing pains along the course of a nerve.

Hand points: Corresponding bodily area point(s).

NEURASTHENIA (neurasthenic neurosis — also see: NERVES; etc.): A group of symptoms which are generally related to nervous exhaustion (e.g., "low energy," weakness, various aches and pains, etc.).

<u>Hand points</u>: See NERVES.

NIGHTMARES (especially affecting children — also see: Dreams, excessive; Hysteria; Nervousness; etc.): Frightening dreams. Primarily a disorder of childhood that passes by age six or seven. Frequent nightmares may indicate need for professional — esp. dietary — counseling.

<u>Hand points</u>: See DREAMING, EXCESSIVE.

NOSE (also see: Nasal congestion; Nosebleed; etc.): The external orifice of the respiratory system. In the traditional Oriental view, the nostrils and nasal passages are controlled by the lungs, while the external part is related to the heart.

<u>Hand points</u>: Nose.

NOSEBLEED (epistaxis — also see: Nose; etc.): A nasal hemorrhage which may be minor and simple or linked to more serious problems such as concussion. <u>Any nosebleed that lasts more than ten or fifteen minutes requires immediate medical attention</u> (since it usually indicates a more serious, underlying condition).

<u>Hand points</u>: A-5; 6; Nose (?).

NUMBNESS: Local or general insensitivity (anesthesia) often coupled with sluggishness, "pins and needles" feeling, tingling, etc. Sudden or unexplained numbness calls for immediate medical attention, since it is usually a symptom of an underlying disorder.

<u>Hand points</u>: (?) Corresponding bodily area points.

OCCIPUT (back of head - also see: Head; Headache; Neck; etc.):

<u>Hand points</u>: Occiput; Neck.

OVARIES (also see: Menstrual difficulites; Sexual organs; etc.): The two female sex glands that germinate egg cells and provide internal secretions (hormones).
   Most common ovarian problems are <u>infections, cysts,</u> tumors and stretching (or straining). When ovarian symptoms occur on the right side, they are easily mistaken for <u>appendicitis.</u> <u>Gonorrhea</u> (as well as tuberculosis) may be particularly harmful to fertility — as well as being a common cause of subsequent arthritis — so any infection of the ovaries or genitourinary system should have prompt, medical attention.

<u>Hand points</u>: Ovary; Uterus; Adrenals.

PAIN CONTROL CENTERS (also see: Headache; Neuralgia; specific portions of body affected, such as Arm; Hand; etc.): Pain is one of the body's first lines of commun- ication and defense and may arise from conditions in parts of the body away from the pain site. For chronic recurring pain, get medical help.

<u>Hand points</u>: Use corresponding bodily area points.

PALATE (also see: MOUTH; etc.): The roof of the mouth, composed of the "hard" and "soft" palates.

<u>Hand points:</u> Mouth; Stomach; Spleen; Pancreas.

PANCREAS (also see: Diabetes; ENDOCRINE GLANDS; Hypoglycemia; SPLEEN; etc.): Located immediately beside the spleen (just behind the bottom of the ribcage and upper abdomen), this gland is responsible for the production of insulin, pancreatic juice, etc. It is a vital organ and is linked, in traditional Oriental theory, to both the spleen and the stomach. It is a prime organ in <u>hypoglycemia</u> (low blood sugar), and problems such as <u>jaundice,</u> <u>diabetes mellitus</u> or <u>pancreatitis</u> may develop from its malfunction. Deep, severe pain between the shoulder blades — especially in middle-aged-to-elderly males — calls for immediate medical attention, since that is a common symptom of pancreatic cancer. (Note: Pancreatitis, on the other hand — an inflammation of the pancreas — affects females more frequently than males.) (For more in-depth techniques for healing this organ, see this author's THE NATURAL HEALER'S ACUPRESSURE HANDBOOK, VOLUME II.)

<u>Hand points:</u> Spleen; Pancreas; Stomach.

PANIC: see FEAR CONTROL CENTERS; HYSTERIA; etc.

PARALYSIS (also see: Numbness; etc.): Loss of sensation and muscle function due to injury to the nervous system and/or disease-linked destruction of the nervous connections. Partial or complete paralysis may even be triggered by psychological problems and conditions such as hysteria. Paralysis may affect specific areas of half the body (hemiplegia) or more. <u>Get medical help</u> <u>immediately.</u> (Note: Paralysis due to <u>brain damage</u> is generally of the <u>stiff</u> or <u>spastic</u> type, whereas spinal disorders generally cause paralysis of the flaccid sort.)

Hand points: Use corresponding bodily area points.

PARASITES, INTERNAL (e.g., pinworms, hookworms, etc.): Symptoms (esp. of worms) often include: Restlessness (esp. at night); nose picking; teeth-grinding or gritting (during sleep); dry cough; anal itching (esp. at night); changes in bowel habits; weight loss or inability to gain weight (esp. tapeworms), etc. Since worms are spread by contact from scratching, food contamination, etc., good hygiene is important. Internal parasites are extremely common, especially in those who keep dogs, cats and other affectionate pets. Numerous allergies or similar problems are parasite-"inspired" (e.g., a common form of asthma appears to arise as a weakened state produced by roundworms, transmitted by dogs).

Hand points: Gastrointestinal.

PARATHYROID GLANDS: See THYROID GLAND. Four tiny bodies on the back of the thyroid gland, which is located in the neck. An important function of the parathyroid glands is to regulate the use of calcium and phosphorus in the body.

PAROTID GLANDS (also see: Mouth; Mumps; Tongue; etc.): The salivary glands found in front of, and below, the (outer) ear. They are shaped like small bunches of grapes.

Hand points: Parotid.

PELVIS: The bony ring formed by the hip bones, the sacrum, the coccyx and the cavity formed by them.

Hand points: (?) Appendix; Prostate.

PERINEUM: That area of the body located between the anus and the sex organs.

Hand points: Perineum.

PERIODONTAL PROBLEMS (e.g., pyorrhea, etc. — also see: Gingivitis; MOUTH; Toothache; etc.): Problems (e.g., inflammation, degeneration, etc.) of the gums and/or bone surrounding the teeth.

Hand points: Mouth; Tooth, teeth.

PERITONITIS (also see: Abdomen, lower; etc.): An inflammation of the wall of the abdominal cavity resulting from any number of sources such as a rup- tured appendix or wound, etc. Its symptoms include severe abdominal pain (often intensified by movement) and abdominal distention. The more severe the problem, the more distended the abdomen may be. Vomiting and/or diarrhea may be present in the early stages; fever, chills, and rapid pulse usually follow. The sufferer appears very sick — which he is.

Peritonitis is a complication of an underlying problem or condition; foods and fluids should not be given. This is an extremely serious problem and, untreated, will usually lead to death. Get medical help immediately.

Hand points: (?) Bladder (urinary); Appendix; Ileo-cecum; Prostate; Uterus.

PHARYNX (also see: Larynx; RESPIRATORY SYSTEM; Throat; Tonsillitis; etc.): The tube that runs from the back of the nose to the esophagus.

Hand points: Throat; Thyroid; Tonsils.

PINEAL GLAND (also see: Brain; Endocrine glands; Head; etc.): A pea-sized gland located near lower part of the brain. While its function is not completely understood, at least one part of its purpose is to deal with the sex organs, their size and development. Like all endocrine glands, its stimulation should only be undertaken with great caution. (Note: Most schools of yoga place high importance on this gland in terms of spiritual and emotional development.)

Hand points: Pineal; Endocrine glands (master point).

PITUITARY GLAND (also see: Endocrine glands; etc.): A vital endocrine gland located near — and attached to — the brain. Like many other endocrine glands, its function is only partially understood. It is a master control for the body's internal secretions (hormones) and is at least partially responsible for sex functions, growth, sexual development, defenses against emergencies and diseases, etc. Stimulate this gland with acupressure cautiously, if at all.

Hand points: Pituitary; Endocrine glands (master point).

PLEURISY (also see: Chest; Pain control centers Pneumonia; etc.): An inflammation of the inner chest cavity sometimes accompanying infections of the lungs and/or chest areas. The primary symptom is pain, either mild or severe, while breathing. Pleurisy is generally symptomatic of a more serious underlying conditon. Get medical help immediately.

Hand points: (?) Chest; Lungs.

PNEUMONIA (also see: Chest; Pleurisy; etc.): An inflammation of the air sacs in the lungs. There are a number of forms of pneumonia, and each represents a potentially dangerous threat. Often pneumonia is a complication of other problems or diseases. Colds and influenza, chronic alcoholism, malnutrition, exposure, and foreign matter in the respiratory tract are only a few of the conditions that may lead to this disorder.
   Although pneumonia may be either bacterial or non-bacterial, symptoms are the same and include shaking chills, sharp pain in either or both sides of the chest, cough with a pinkish-to-rusty sputum, fever and headache. Get medical help immediately.

Hand points: (?) Chest; Lungs.

PROSTATE (also see: Sexual organs; etc.): The organ surrounding the neck of the urinary bladder in the male. Symptoms of prostate problems often include itching and burning in and around the front of the urethral canal (urethral meatus) of the penis, especially in the morning, and pain in the groin and/or lower back region.

Hand points: Prostate; Bladder (urinary) (?).

PSORIASIS (also see: SKIN; etc.): A chronic, inflammatory skin and scalp disorder characterized by reddened patches covered with silvery white scales. This disorder tends to run in families and usually occurs after a strep infection, skin injury, emotional shock or stressful situation. It is not contagious, infectious or particularly uncomfortable. It is more common in people who drink large amounts of liquor.

Hand points: See SKIN.

RECTUM (also see: Gastrointestinal system; Gonorrhea; Hemorrhoids; etc.): The lowest part of the large intestine, ending at the anus.

Hand points: Rectum.

RESPIRATORY SYSTEM (also see: Bronchitis; Chest; Lungs; Pneumonia; etc.): The system of the body pertaining to the breathing apparatus. This includes the nasal cavities; pharynx; larynx; trachea; bronchi; broncheoles; and the lungs (primary organs, in traditional Oriental theory, which are paired with the colon).

The most common problem to this system — and one of man's most common health problems — is the "common" cold (upper respiratory infection). Other problems include: Pneumonia; tuberculosis; emphysema; allergic reactions (e.g, "hay fever," sneezing, coughing, etc.); and, less commonly, such problems as celiac disease ("sprue" or gluten allergy), etc.

Hand points: Adrenals; Colon (all); Lung.

RETCHING: See VOMITING AND RETCHING.

RHEUMATISM: See bodily area affected, such as
SHOULDER, etc.

RHINITIS: See ALLERGIES; HAY FEVER; NASAL
CONGESTION; SINUSITIS.

SCAPULA (shoulder blade — also see: Back, upper;
etc.): The large triangular bones located in the upper
back, to either side of the spine.

Hand points: See BACK, UPPER.

SCIATICA (also see: Back, lower; Buttocks; HIP;
NEURALGIA; Leg; Lumbago; Pain control centers etc.):
Pain and tenderness along the sciatic nerve, ranging
from the lower back down (distally) as far as the foot.
Sciatica differs from "normal" back pain in that the
pain usually radiates from the lower back down the rear
portion of the leg (vs. being localized in the back
alone).

Hand points: (?) Sciatic nerve; Hip; Nerves.

SEASICKNESS (also see: Dizziness; Vertigo; Vomiting and
retching; etc.): A minor-to-severe feeling of illness,
nausea and queasiness, often accompanied by vomiting
and retching, dizziness, loss of appetite, etc. It is
primarily associated with the motion of a boat or ship
at sea, but may be triggered by the rocking of an
unstable platform. While this unpleasant condition
might last as long as several days in an unstable site,

it is usually only a temporary problem that eases as one's equilibrium becomes more attuned to the surrounding environment or as soon as one reaches a firm, stable location. Drink no alcohol. In traditional Oriental theory, seasickness — and other forms of motion illness — are symptoms of liver disorder (which helps explain why seasick sufferers actually turn greenish — one indication of extreme liver and/or gallbladder distress). Seasickness is more prevalent during the day — especially on foggy days — than at night.

Hand points: (?) Gastrointestinal; Liver; Gallbladder; Ear (inner).

SEXUAL DRIVE (also see: FRIGIDITY; Genitourinary system; IMPOTENCE; Sexual organs; etc.): Problems with the sexual drive (libido or primal-pleasure drive) are of one of two types: Being "too hot"; or being "too cold."

"Too hot" is characterized by strong interest or aversion to sexual activity, to the point that it becomes a problem (e.g., too much activity, thought and/or fantasy directed toward sexual fullment, real or imagined, on a regular basis). This is caused primarily by "extreme" foods.

"Too cold" is characterized by little or no interest in sexual activity, impotence, etc., which is generally caused by disease (e.g., diabetes), drugs (e.g., certain hypertensives, etc.) or such dietary problems as malnutrition, alcoholism, etc. Sexual drive is primarily a "child" of the kidneys, liver and heart. Any problems with these organs may reflect themselves in the sexual drive. Further information about "balancing" the sexual drive may be found in this author's HOW TO ENJOY SEX MORE WITH ACUGENICS (available through the G-Jo Institute).

Hand points: See FRIGIDITY; IMPOTENCE.

SEXUAL ORGANS (also see: GENITOURINARY SYSTEM;
Sexual drive; Vaginitis; Gonorrhea; Prostate; etc.):
Includes the penis, testicles and related parts of the
male reproductive system; and the vagina, ovaries, and
womb (uterus) of the female system. The sexual organs
develop from — and are "children" of — the kidneys
(and urinary bladder) in traditional Oriental theory.
  Common problems of the sexual organs include:
Gonorrhea (see GONORRHEA); herpes simplex II virus
(see HERPES); vaginal yeast infections (see VAGINITIS);
infections; pain in/around sexual organs; sterility/
infertility (see FERTILITY); discharges; slow maturity;
etc.

Hand points: Ovary; Sex organs; Testicles; Uterus.

SHINGLES (HERPES ZOSTER) — also see: Bodily area
affected): A particularly painful infection of the
central nervous system. Its symptoms include small
eruptions and neuralgic pain, especially around the
waist. Shingles most often occurs in persons over
fifty-years-old.

Hand points: Chest; Waist (?).

SHOULDER (also see: NECK, etc.):

Hand points: Shoulder; Arm (?).

SINUSITIS (problems of the sinuses — also see:
Headache; Nasal congestion; etc.): Inflammation of the
sinus cavities in and around the nose and eyes. When an

acupressure point is stimulated, there may be drainage. Sinusitis is an allergic reaction — much like hay fever (allergic rhinitis) — that is "triggered" by certain dietary, emotional and/or environmental phenomena but whose "stage is set" by continued abusive practices (usually dietary). It is primarily a problem of the kidneys, adrenals, lungs and colon (large intestine), in traditional Oriental theory. It may also be related to thyroid dysfunction and/or tooth infection.

Hand points: (?) Lungs; Nose; Sinuses; Kidneys; Adrenals.

SKIN (also see: Acne; etc.): In traditional Oriental theory, the skin is a "child" of the lungs and colon. A problem of the skin often also indicates an imbalanced state with the kidneys. Conversely, as the kidneys and/or lungs and colon return to balance, the skin clears. Skin problems may also indicate a thyroid dysfunction.

Hand points: Lungs; Colon (all); Kidneys; Bladder (urinary); Thyroid (use cautiously).

SMALL INTESTINE (also see: GASTROINTESTINAL SYSTEM; HEART; Ulcers, intestinal; etc.): The primary organ — "mated" with heart, in traditional Oriental theory — which connects the bottom of the stomach with the beginning of the colon (large intestine). The small intestine has three parts — the duodenum, the jejunum and ileium — and serves, among others, the functions of creating sludge from the stomach contents and several blood-related chores. (For more in-depth techniques for healing this organ, see THE NATURAL HEALER'S ACUPRESSURE HANDBOOK, VOLUME II.)

Hand points: (?) Gastrointestinal; Heart.

SNORING: During sleep, breathing in such a way as to rattle and vibrate the soft palate (usually when sleeping on back). May arise from "sleep apnea" (or "forgetting" to breathe for prolonged periods of time), and is most common in overweight males with short necks. (Note: Have victim — the person kept awake — try triggering points gently when snorer is snoring.)

Hand points: (?) Nose.

SOLAR PLEXUS (celiac plexus): The region — especially the nerve network — extending downward from the area of the heart into the upper abdomen.

Hand points: Solar plexus.

SORES (on skin — also see: Boils, styes, carbuncles; Skin; etc.): Skin disorders and eruptions, these are often symptoms of disorder in the genitourinary system. Any slow-healing, returning or otherwise suspicious sore — especially on the face, ears, hands, lower forearms and/or lower legs (common sites for skin cancer to develop) — should have prompt medical attention.

Hand points: Use corresponding bodily area points.

SORE THROAT: See Colds and influenza; Throat; etc.

SPASM, MUSCULAR: See CRAMPS and SPASMS, MUSCULAR; MUSCLES; PAIN.

SPINAL CORD (also see: Back, lower and upper; NERVES; Vertebrae; etc.): That part of the central nervous system carried within the spinal column.

Hand points: (?) Nerves; Spinal cord.

SPLEEN (also see: Diabetes mellitus; Gallbladder; Liver; Pancreas; Stomach; etc.): Located in the upper left-hand quarter of the abdomen, beneath or behind the left side of the ribcage, the spleen is the largest lymph gland of the body. In traditional Oriental theory, it is paired with or "mated" (along with the pancreas) to the stomach and is a primary organ. The spleen is the central organ of the lymph system, whose chore is (among other functions) the cleansing of impurities from the blood.

Splenic problems may manifest themselves as pain in the left side radiating up to the shoulder, hot and dry skin, thirst, possibly dark and scanty urine, constipation, etc. It is the primary organ affected by diabetes, in the traditional Oriental theory.

The spleen is also vital in the process of controlling disease. Because of its close connection with the lymph system, it is important in the blood-cleansing and circulating process. Thus it is a primarily affected organ in such disorders as: Hodgkin's disease; leukemia; anemia; septicemia; etc.

The spleen is subject to such phenomena as enlargement or rupture as well as inflammation. In Western medical theory, the spleen is not considered essential and is removed by surgery regularly; in traditional Oriental theory, on the other, it (in conjunction with the pancreas) is one of the twelve most important organs and is responsible for many functions of maintenance, both physical and emotional. (For more in-depth techniques for healing this organ, see this author's THE NATURAL HEALER'S ACUPRESSURE HANDBOOK, VOLUME II.)

Hand points Spleen; Stomach; Pancreas; D-19, 20.

SPRAINS, MUSCULAR (also see: Muscles; Pain control centers Strains, muscular; specific areas of injury, such as Foot, Wrist, etc.): Injuries to the soft tissues surrounding the joints. Sprains generally occur when the joint is forced into more extreme action than it is capable of handling. Keep stress away from the sprained area since the injury is sometimes a tearing or partial ripping of the ligaments, muscles and/or blood vessels of the affected area.

Hand points: Use corresponding bodily area points.

STOMACH (also see: Abdomen, upper; Gallbladder; Gastrointestinal system; Indigestion; etc.): This dilated organ of the gastrointestinal system is located directly below the diaphragm. In traditional Oriental theory, the stomach is the organic "mate" of the spleen (and pancreas), and is a primary organ of digestion whose major physical function is breaking down and dissolving food. (Note: Pain arising soon after eating usually indicates trouble in upper stomach — especially a stomach ulcer — and is often caused by excessive sweet/sugary foods; pain that is relieved by eating may indicate a duodenal ulcer). (For more in-depth techniques for healing this organ, see this author's THE NATURAL HEALER'S ACU-PRESSURE HANDBOOK, VOLUME II.)

Hand points: See GASTROINTESTINAL SYSTEM; Digestion; Spleen (?); Pancreas (?); Stomach; D-18.

STONES, GALLBLADDER: See GALLSTONES.

STONES, KIDNEY or BLADDER (urolithiases — also see GENITOURINARY SYSTEM; KIDNEYS; etc.): Calculi formed from normal constituents of urine which have combined into a relatively insoluble crystalline substance by whatever deficiencies or imbalances that exist to precipitate them. There are several different kinds of kidney stones. May be associated with gout and symptomatic of incomplete protein absorption or assimilation. Kidney stones occur equally between both sexes, while bladder stones are far more frequent in males. Pain is likely to be excruciating — esp. in the flanks (area between ribs and hips) — if the stone(s) pass from the kidneys. Get medical help immediately. And since stones are of several types, if it passes out of the system, collect it for laboratory examination.

Hand points: (?) Kidneys; Bladder (urinary).

STRAINS, MUSCULAR (including "charley horse" — also see: Muscles; Pain control centers Sprains, muscular; etc.): Muscular strains are much like sprains, except they usually occur away from the joint. With muscular strains, muscle fibers are stretched too far, sometimes even torn. Strains commonly occur in the lower back, triggered by improper lifting or hoisting. In short, they are muscle injuries due to improper or over-exertion.

<u>Hand points</u>: Muscles; plus corresponding bodily area points.

STYES: See BOILS, STYES, CARBUNCLES.

SWEATING CONTROL CENTERS: The primary function of sweating is to regulate the body's temperature; as moisture evaporates, cooling occurs. Normally, about a pint to one and a half pints of perspiration (a usually acid fluid, comprised of about 99% water plus urea and various salts) are lost each day. Before using acupressure-point stimulation, relax for a few minutes especially if sweating has been produced by hard, physical labor or exercise. (Note: Perspiration has a diagnostic quality as well: If your perspiration tastes salty, you may be using too much salt in your diet).

<u>Hand points</u>: D-15, 16.

SWELLING (also see: Edema; Sprains, muscular; Strains, muscular; etc.): A non-specific accumulation of fluid in various tissues. Since swelling without injury may be symptomatic of potentially serious underlying health problems, get medical attention for this problem.

<u>Hand points</u>: Use corresponding bodily area points.

TACHYCARDIA, PAROXYSMAL (also see: Fear; Heart; Hysteria; etc.): A condition when the heartbeat rate suddenly and dramatically increases. An attack may last from minutes to days, stopping as suddenly as it began. It may be associated with heart disease, but not necessarily. There may or may not be pain. Get medical help immediately.

Hand points: E-17.

TENNIS ELBOW: See ELBOW.

TESTICLES, INCLUDING CRUSHED TESTICLES (also see: Pain control centers Sexual organs; etc.): Injury to the testicles is one of the most painful and agonizing conditions that can happen to the male body; even a mild injury to the testicles may be completely debilitating.

Hand points: Sex organs; Testicles.

TETANUS (lockjaw — also see: Bites, animal, human and insect;): An infectious disease caused by a wound not exposed to oxygen. Any wound may result in tetanus infection; punctures and bites are notorious, especially where there is the presence of rust and/or fecal matter.

As tetanus progresses, spasms of the voluntary muscles occur and convulsions become frequent. Muscle stiffness after a puncture wound (any time between two and 50 days, but usually between five and 10 days) should lead you to suspect tetanus, especially if you have had no inoculation against the disease within several years.

With tetanus, the jaw muscles will eventually lock, accompanied by a grotesque grimace or smile with raised eyebrows. Untreated tetanus is generally fatal. For any wound, if you have not had a recent tetanus vaccination, get medical help immediately.

Hand points: Use corresponding bodily area points;
Nerves.

THIGH (also see: Hip; Knee; Leg; Pain): The part of the
leg from the pelvis to the knee.

Hand points: Leg (?);

THROAT (also see: Colds and influenza; Hoarseness;
Laryngitis; Larynx; PHARYNX; RESPIRATORY SYSTEM;
Tonsillitis; etc.): In traditional Oriental theory,
the throat is primarily associated with the lungs and
colon, and secondarily with the kidneys and urinary
bladder.

Hand points: Throat; Lungs (?).

THYMUS GLAND (also see: Endocrine glands; etc.): An
endocrine gland, located in the chest near the heart.
It is normal for this gland to be most active during
the first year of life, then to atrophy to virtual
non-existence. However, its effects are apparently felt
throughout life, affecting primarily the sex glands,
metabolism of calcium and in early years, the
development of the skeleton. (Note: Any self-treatment
of the endocrine glands should be done with moderation,
if at all.)

Hand points: (?) Thymus.

THYROID GLAND (including Parathyroid gland — also
see: Endocrine glands; Pharynx; etc.): One of the most
vital endocrine glands, problems of the thyroid —
which is located in the front part of the throat, along

the windpipe (pharynx) — are often associated with diabetic or pre-diabetic conditions. Other conditions reflected/caused by dysfunctioning thyroid include: Goiter; certain heart disorders; "pop-eyed" (Graves) disease; cretinism; etc.

Common symptoms of imbalanced thyroid activity include: Cold feet; low energy; poor growth (in children); arrhythmia; sexual difficulties; heat intolerance; dry skin; chapped lips; coarse skin; nervousness; weight imbalances; goiter; etc. (Note: Any self-treatment of the endocrine glands should be done with moderation, if at all.)

Hand points: Thyroid (and parathyroid); Throat; Endocrine glands (master point).

TINNITUS (also see: EAR; HEARING DIFFICULTIES; etc.): A disorder of the inner ear characterized by a ringing sensation, often coupled with dizziness, may be a result of high blood pressure, glandular disorder, ear wax, etc. It is often an early symptom of Meniere's Syndrome.

Hand points: Ear; Kidneys; Bladder (urinary); Eustachian tubes; Vertebrae.

TOES: See ATHLETE'S FOOT; FOOT.

TONGUE (also see: MOUTH; Tonsillitis; etc.): In traditional Oriental theory, the tongue — which functions as the primary "sub-organ" of taste, speech and swallowing — is a "child" of the heart and is also closely associated with the stomach. Thus, ailments of the tongue may indicate imbalance of one or both those major organs.

<u>Hand points</u>: Mouth.

TONSILLITIS (also see: Throat; PANCREAS; PHARYNX;
SPLEEN; Stomach; etc.): Inflammation of the tonsils
(small glands in the throat). Symptoms include
chills, soreness, rapidly rising temperature,
difficulty in swallowing, stiff neck, etc.
　In traditional Oriental theory, the tonsils are
related to the spleen (and pancreas) and stomach.
Abuses to these organs quickly "reflect" themselves in
inflammation of the tonsils (if you are prone to
tonsillitis). (Note: After tonsillectomies — removal
of tonsils — people run a higher risk of lymph cancer
— called Hodgkin's Disease — and multiple sclerosis.
On the other hand, complications of tonsillitis may
include scarlet fever, sinusitis, ear infections,
quinsy — a peritonsillar abscess — and, rarely,
arthritis or meningitis.)

<u>Hand points</u>: Occiput; Throat; Tonsils; C-15.

TOOTH, TEETH (including GUMS — also see: Dental
work; Jaw, lower, upper; MOUTH; TOOTHACHE; etc.):
In traditional Oriental theory, the teeth are
considered primarily as "children" of the colon (large
intestine).
　Common problems of the teeth and gums include:
Decay (cavities or dental caries); spongy gums;
receding gums; infection and toothache; bruxism (or
tooth-grinding, esp. during sleep). Cavities and
pyorrhea (a gum disease) seldom occur in the same
mouth.

<u>Hand points</u>: Tooth, teeth; Mouth.

TOOTHACHE (also see: DENTAL WORK; TOOTH, TEETH, etc.): Pain in the nerve of a tooth, usually caused by infection or inflammation arising from dental caries (cavities). Since gums are essential parts of the tooth system, a problem in these soft tissues which cover the alveolar bone may also be the source of tooth problems.

Abscesses (pods of infection, usually at the bases of teeth) may directly or indirectly affect the heart, lungs, liver, gallbladder, stomach or kidneys (at least) — usually depending on the specific tooth affected — so it is important to seek prompt medical/dental attention for any toothache.

Hand points: Throat; Mouth; Tooth, teeth.

TOOTH EXTRACTION, DRILLING, etc.: See DENTAL WORK.

TORTICOLLIS (stiff neck, "wry neck"): See NECK; WHIPLASH (neck injury).

TRACHEA (also see: Larynx; Respiratory system; Throat; etc.): The windpipe extending from the larynx to the bronchi.

Hand points: (?) Throat; Tonsils; Lungs.

TRAVEL SICKNESS (also see: Dizziness; SEASICKNESS; Vertigo; etc.): A general term for the symptoms that arise from motion and instability. The inner ear and the liver are the primarily affected bodily area and organ.

<u>Hand points</u>: See SEASICKNESS.

"TRAVELER'S DIARRHEA" (see DYSENTERY):
A mild-to-moderate form of amoebic dysentery often
encountered when traveling to warm, primitive
countries.

TRIGEMINAL NEURALGIA (tic doloureaux — also see:
Face; Nerves; Neuralgia; etc.): A particularly painful
form of facial neuralgia that generally begins in
middle life and occurs more frequently in females than
males. Both the intensity of pain and frequency (as
well as duration) of attacks tend to increase. Seizures
appear to occur more frequently in spring and fall as
well as near the changes of season.

<u>Hand points</u>: <u>Throat</u>; (?) Eye; Nerves; Ear.

ULCERS (digestive — also see: Abdomen, upper;
GASTROINTESTINAL SYSTEM; Stomach; etc.): Lesions
that form in the digestive tract and are often associated with stress. There are several types, depending in
which section of the gastrointestinal system they form:
    1. Stomach (gastric) ulcer — characterized by a
"sluggish" stomach (from underproduction of stomach
acids) that is <u>aggravated</u> by eating;
    2. Intestinal (duodenal) ulcers — characterized by
"hunger" pains that are <u>relieved</u> — and stay relieved
for several hours — by eating.
    Ulcer symptoms tend to peak in spring and fall,
with bleeding from an ulcer being most common in
January and September.

<u>Hand points</u>: See GASTROINTESTINAL SYSTEM;
Gastrointestinal.

ULCERS, ORAL ("thrush," canker sores, "trench mouth," etc. — also see: MOUTH; etc.): Lesions which develop from fungus infections, ususally in infants or elderly people. These are often accompanied by fever, gastrointestinal distress and the infection may spread to other parts of the body (e.g., buttocks, groin, etc.).

Hand points: See MOUTH; D-18, 19.

ULCERS, SKIN (also see: Diabetes; SKIN; Varicose veins; etc.): Nearly always, ulcers (and similar lesions) of the skin arise from an underlying health problem (e.g., diabetes mellitus, varicose veins, etc.). Get immediate medical attention for any ulceration (or similar deep sores) of the skin.

Hand points: See SKIN.

URETERS, URETER TUBES (also see: Bladder, urinary; GENITOURINARY SYSTEM; Kidneys; etc.): The long, slender tubes leading/carrying urine from the kidneys to the urinary bladder.

Hand points: See GENITOURINARY SYSTEM.

URETHRA (also see: Bladder, urinary; GENITOURINARY SYSTEM; etc.): The tube (longer on males, shorter in females) leading from the urinary bladder to carry urine out of the body. (Note: Any urethritis — infection of the urethra — may be symptomatic of a venereal disease, such as gonorrhea, etc.; if this is suspected, get medical help immediately.)

Hand points: See GENITOURINARY SYSTEM; F-18, 19.

URINARY CONTROL CENTERS (also see: Cystitis; Genitourinary system; Stones, kidney or bladder; etc.): To help bring temporary relief (up to half an hour or so) from the need to   urinate. This technique may be helpful in a situation where facilities are not immediately available, as in driving, etc. Frequent urination (more than six times daily for a male or seven times daily for a female) on a prolonged basis (beyond a short stressful period in life, say) may require professional attention.

Hand points: F-18, 19 (esp. nocturia — frequency of urination at night); Bladder (urinary); Kidneys (?).

UTERUS (womb — also see GENITOURINARY SYSTEM; Sexual organs; etc.): The three-inch long, thick walled female reproductive organ that receives and holds the (fertilized) egg which develops into the fetus. If the egg is not fertilized, then the lining is shed each month (menstruation).

Hand points: Uterus; Sex organs.

VAGINITIS (vaginal yeast infection, etc. — also see: Cystitis; GENITOURINARY SYSTEM; Sexual organs; etc.): A very common female ailment sometimes transmitted by males through sexual intercourse. Its symptoms — commonly abnormal itching, burning, discharge, etc. — may mask more serious problems, especially syphilis, gonorrhea, etc. For this reason — and because your sexual partner(s) may need treatment — seek medical advice if this condition is suspected.

Yeast (candida, monilia) is a common cause of vaginitis, as are trichomonas and other parasites or bacteria. Diabetes, pregnancy and taking birth control pills are also important possible factors in this condition.

The following "self-diagnosis" may be helpful in identifying the type of vaginal infection you are suffering:

Yeast — produces thick, white, creamy and/or curd-like discharge (usually odorless but with intense itching and/or burning/soreness). This condition often occurs in pregnancy and diabetes as a result of contraceptives, etc.

Bacterial — produces a watery, gray-to-white discharge that may by foul-smelling, but is seldom accompanied by much physical discomfort.

Non-Specific — produces a foul-smelling discharge (and may arise from a combination of bacteria). (Note: Vaginitis may be a symptom of gonorrhea or other sexually transmittable disease — if this is suspected, get medical help immediately).

Hand points: See GENITOURINARY, SEX ORGANS.

VARICOSE VEINS: Swollen, inflamed/enlarged veins, most often found on the inner and/or back side of the calf and inner thigh. They are most often the shallower (vs. deeper) veins — those which are less supported by muscles.

Varicose veins may be caused by such problems as phlebitis, pregnancy (or other excessive weight/ pressure on the abdomen), etc. Ulceration may occur in advanced cases. (Note: Varicose veins may be a precursor of thrombophlebitis — a dangerous condition; get medical attention for any varicose veins, or for symptoms of aching, burning, itching and/or pain, especially in the legs.)

<u>Hand points</u>: Liver; Kidneys.

VERTEBRAE/S (also see: Back, lower and/or upper;
etc.): The 33 bones forming the vertebral (spinal)
column. This column is "divided" into "sections":
<u>Cervical</u> (highest — from the head to the shoulder
area); <u>Thoracic</u> (central — from the top rib to the
lowest rib); <u>Lumbar</u> (lower — from the bottom rib
downward); <u>Sacral</u> (sacrum — the triangular "bone"
at the bottom of the spine, just above the coccyx,
comprised of five fused vertebrae).

<u>Hand points</u>: Vertebrae.

VERTIGO (also see: DIZZINESS; Seasickness; Travel
sickness; etc.): True vertigo is a sensation/ feeling
that the outer world is revolving about the sufferer
(as may occur with intoxication) or that he himself is
moving in some disoriented space. However, vertigo is
more commonly (and erroneously) used to mean dizziness,
giddiness, lightheadedness, etc. Vertigo may also be
accompanied by ringing in the ears (tinnitus) and/or
rapid, uncontrolled eye movements (nystagmus).

<u>Hand points</u>: Head.

VITILIGO (also see: SKIN; etc.): A disorder of the skin
pigmentation in which pigmentation (skin coloring)
disappears, leaving spots or patches of white. While
spontaneous repigmentation may occur, it is rare. The
disorder is probably related to a dysfunction of the
lungs and/or kidneys (in traditional Oriental theory).
While repigmentation is unlikely, the disorder may be
slowed with the acupressure techniques.

Hand points: Use corresponding bodily area points
(?).

VOMITING AND RETCHING (also see: Stomach; etc.):
Symptomatic of many problems, and not all of them
associated with the digestive tract. Dehydration is
always a problem with continued loss of fluids; if
vomiting is severe, get medical help immediately.
(Note: It is vital to prevent dehydration, especially
in the very young, the elderly and the seriously ill or
injured. Feed Gatorade® or similar fluid replacer —
if not available, use one qt. of boiled water plus
juice of four oranges plus seven tsp. of white sugar
plus one tsp. of salt; sip, medicinally. Also if there
is repeated vomiting/nausea after head injury, medical
attention is imperative).

Hand points: Chest; Stomach (?).

WHIPLASH (neck injury—also see: Neck; Pain control
centers etc.): A condition that may occur when the neck
is snapped suddenly forward or back, as in the event of
an automobile accident. Get medical help immediately.

Hand points: (?) Neck.

WRIST (including carpal tunnel syndrome, sprain, etc.
— also see: Hand; etc.):

Hand points: Wrist.

SECTION II

HAND ACUPRESSURE POINTS:
THEIR LOCATIONS AND USES

REMINDER: The acupressure points in the following pages are approximate. They represent a compilation of the opinions of many authorities in the field of acupressure plus the author's own experience. The precise location of your own points will be determined by finding the most pressure-sensitive spots in the general areas described and illustrated in the following pages.

ALSO: In the following pages you may find an acupressure point preceded — or followed — by a question mark (?). This is meant to indicate an unacknowledged (by other authorities in the field) but probable location, based on the author's experience and/or acupressure theory.

NAME OF HAND POINT	LOCATION OF HAND POINT
Adrenals	D-17, 19, 20; E-16
Ankle	A-4
Anus	C-14, 15; D-14
Appendix	E-14 (right hand only)
Arm	B-3
Bladder (urinary)	C-14; D-14, 15; E-14
Brain	A-17
Chest	A-6; B-17
Coccyx	D-14
Colon (general)	C-20
Colon, ascending	D-15 (right hand only); E-14, 15 (right hand)
Colon, descending	D-15 (left hand only); E-14, 15 (left hand)
Colon, Sigmoid	See Sigmoid colon, flexure
Colon, transverse	C-15, 16; D-15, 16; E-16

Digestion (food)	B-15, 16; C-14
Ear	E-17, 18; F-18, 19, 20
Ear, inner (hearing)	E-19, 20, 21, 22; F-19, 20
Endocrine glands (master points)	D-19, 20
Eustachian tubes	B-18; C-18
Eye	A-7, 17; B-17; C-19, 20, 21; D-18, 19, 20, 21, 22
Forehead	B-8, 9
Gallbladder	D-16 (right hand only); E-16 (right hand), E-19 (?); F-16 (right hand only)
Gastrointestinal	D-16; E-15
Head	A-17, 18; B-5; F-17 (skull)
Heart	C-15, 17 (left hand only); D-17 (left hand only), D-21; E-16 (left hand); F-15, 16, 17
Heel	D-14
Hip	E-14; F-14
Hypothalamus	A-17
Ileo-cecum	E-15 (right hand only)
Intestine, small	B-15; C-15, 19; D-15; E-15

Kidneys	D-17; E-15, 16, 17
Leg	C-5; D-5
Liver	D-16 (right side only); E-16 (right side only), E-17, 19; F-16 (right side only), F-17
Lungs	C-17; D-16, 17, 18; E-17
Mastoid	F-17
Mental powers, facilities	A-18; B-18
Mouth	D-18
Muscles; muscular strength	C-15, 16, 19, 20, 21; D-19, 20, 21, 22
Neck	A-17; B-7, 15, 16, 17; C-7
Nerves	A-17, 18; B-15, 16, 17, 18; C-19, 20, 21; D-19, 20, 21, 22
Nose	B-5; C-18
Occiput (back of head)	E-7; F-7
Ovary	E-13, 14
Pancreas	D-16 (left hand only), D-17; E-16, 17, E-20, 21 (left hand only)
Parotid	F-18

Perineum	E-8
Pineal	A-18
Pituitary	A-18
Prostate	C-13
Rectum	C-14, 15; D-14
Sciatic nerve	D-6, 7
Sex organs	C-13; D-14; E-14
Shoulder	B-7; F-15
Sigmoid colon, flexure	E-14 (left hand only)
Sinuses	C-18; D-18; E-18; F-18
Solar plexus	C-17
Spinal cord	C-14, 15, 16, 17; E-6
Spleen	D-16 (left hand only); E-15, 16 (left hand only), E-20, 21 (left hand ?); F-15 (left hand only)
Stomach	C-16, 17; D-16
Testicles	E-13
Throat	B-16; C-7, 16; D-7
Thymus	C-18; D-17, 18
Thyroid and parathyroid	C-15, 16, 18

Tonsils	C-17, 18
Tooth; teeth	D-18
Uterus	C-13
Vertebrae	C-5; D-5, 13; E-13
Waist	C-5; D-5
Wrist	C-4

Blank chart — make notes here...

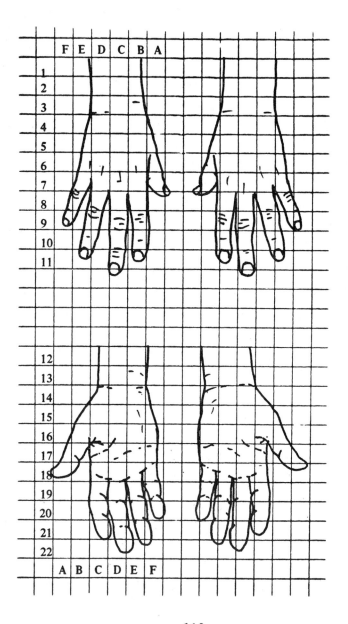

NAME OF HAND POINT: Adrenals

LOCATION OF POINT: D–17, 19, 20; E-16

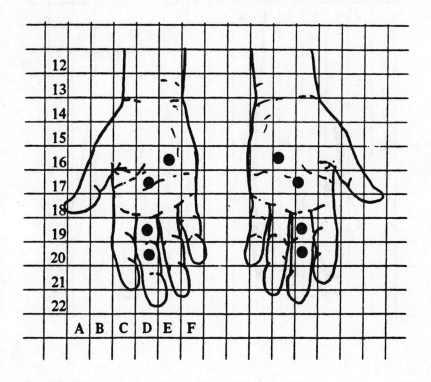

NAME OF HAND POINT: Ankle

LOCATION OF POINT: A-4

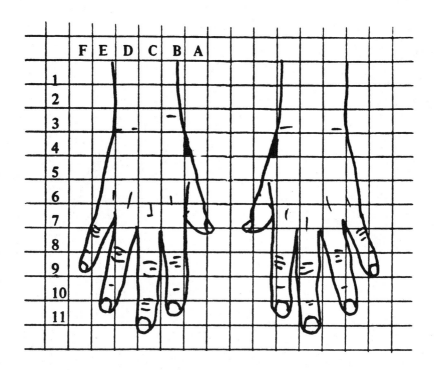

NAME OF HAND POINT: Anus

LOCATION OF POINT: C-14, 15; D-14

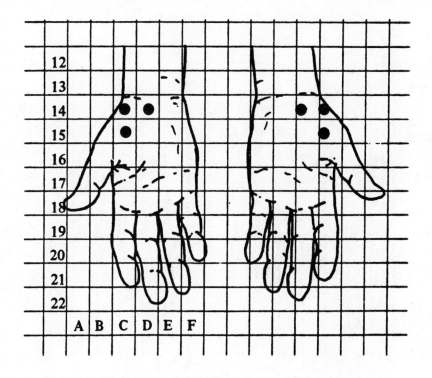

NAME OF HAND POINT: Appendix

LOCATION OF POINT: E-14 (right hand only)

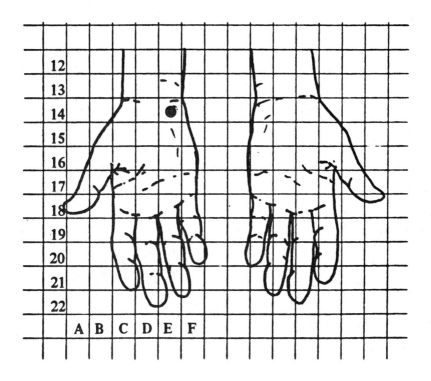

NAME OF HAND POINT: Arm

LOCATION OF POINT: B-3

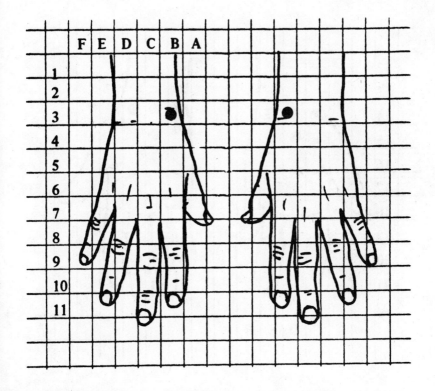

NAME OF HAND POINT: Bladder (urinary)

LOCATION OF POINT: C-14; D-14, 15; E-14

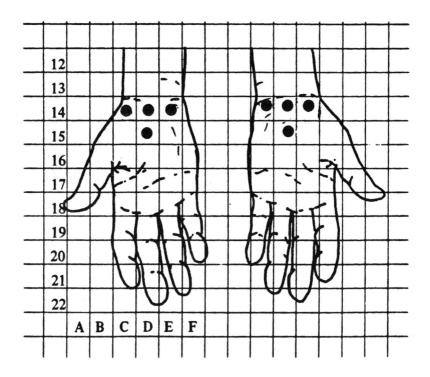

NAME OF HAND POINT: Brain

LOCATION OF POINT: A-17

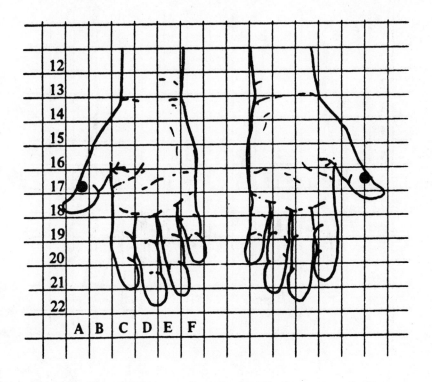

NAME OF HAND POINT: Chest

LOCATION OF POINT: A-6

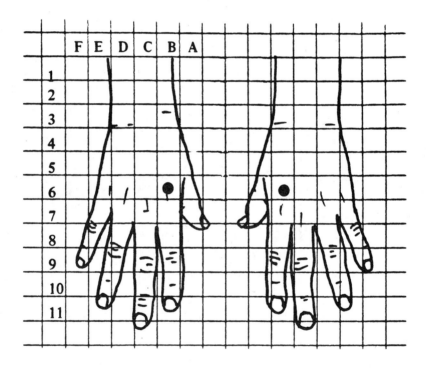

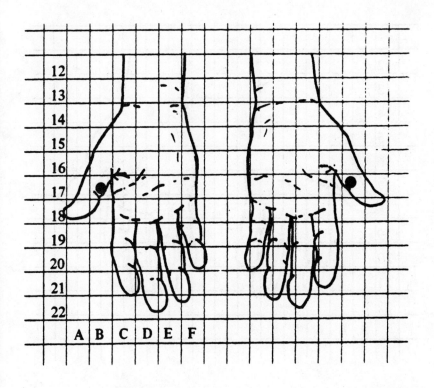

NAME OF HAND POINT: Coccyx

LOCATION OF POINT: D-14

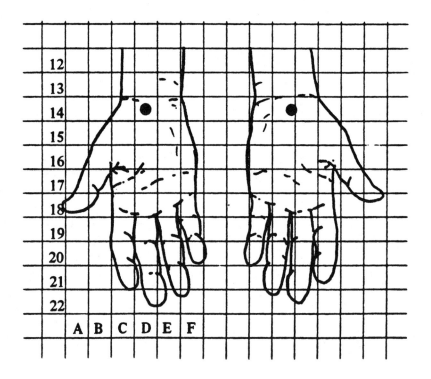

NAME OF HAND POINT: Colon (general)

LOCATION OF POINT: C-20

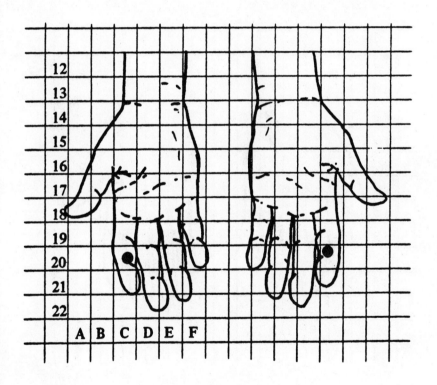

NAME OF HAND POINT: Colon, ascending

LOCATION OF POINT: D–15 (right hand only); E-14, 15
(right hand)

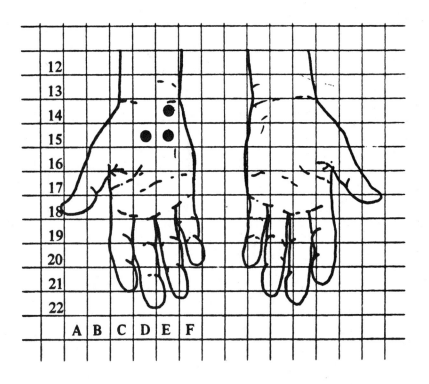

NAME OF HAND POINT: Colon, descending

LOCATION OF POINT: D-15 (left hand only); E-14, 15 (left hand)

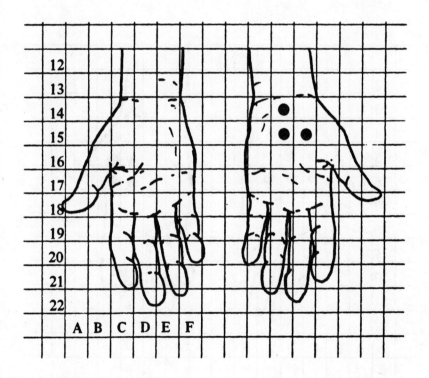

NAME OF HAND POINT: Colon, transverse

LOCATION OF POINT: C-15, 16; D-15, 16; E-16

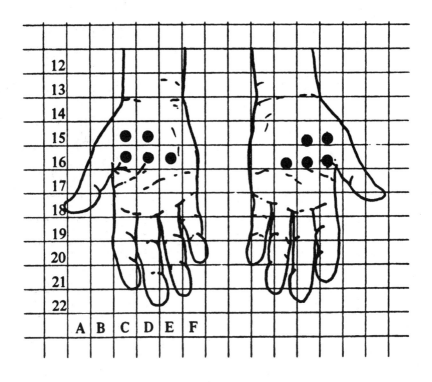

NAME OF HAND POINT: Digestion (food)

LOCATION OF POINT: B-15, 16; C-14

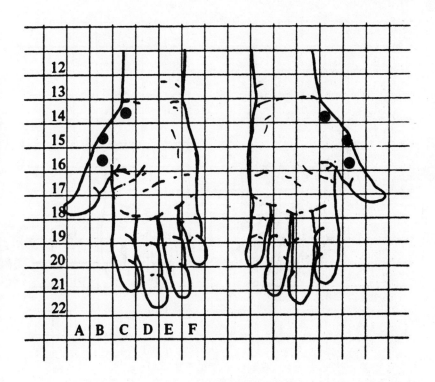

NAME OF HAND POINT: Ear

LOCATION OF POINT: E-17, 18; F-18, 19, 20

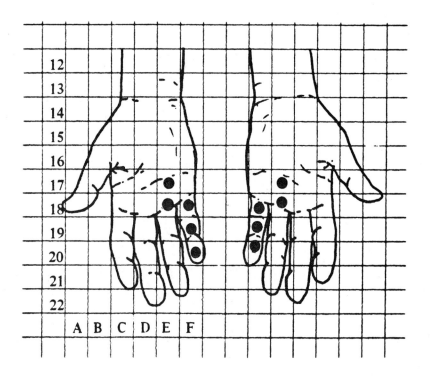

NAME OF HAND POINT: Ear, inner (hearing)

LOCATION OF POINT: E-19, 20, 21, 22; F-19, 20

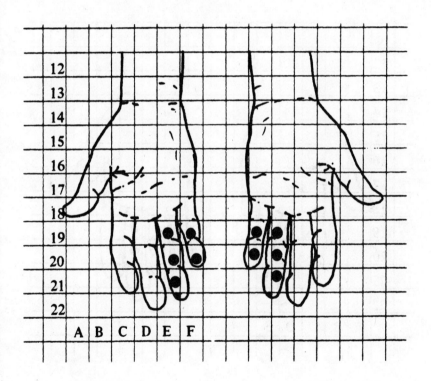

NAME OF HAND POINT: Endocrine glands

LOCATION OF POINT: D-19, 20

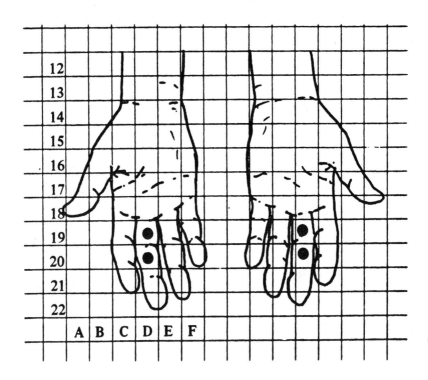

NAME OF HAND POINT: Eustachian tubes

LOCATION OF POINT: B-18; C-18

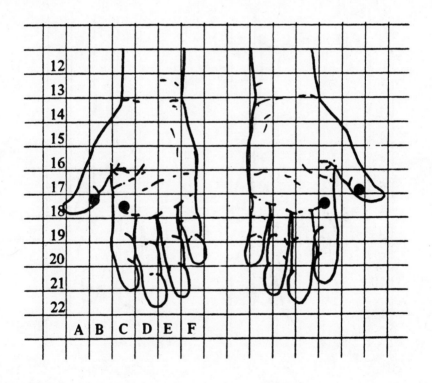

NAME OF HAND POINT: Eye

LOCATION OF POINT: A-7

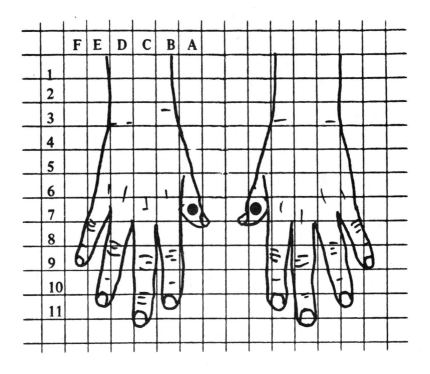

NAME OF HAND POINT: Eye continued...

LOCATION OF POINT: A-17; B-17; C-19, 20, 21; D-18, 19, 20, 21, 22

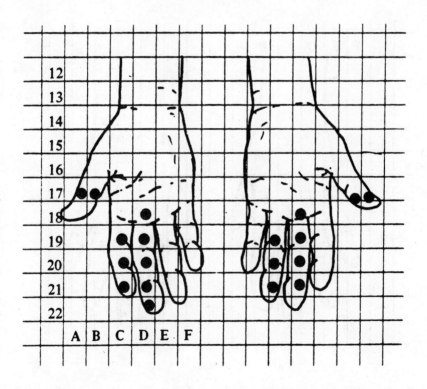

NAME OF HAND POINT: Forehead

LOCATION OF POINT: B-8, 9

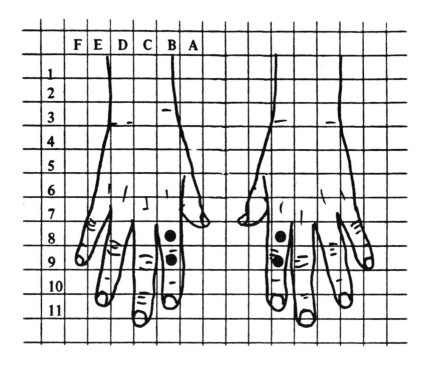

NAME OF HAND POINT: Gallbladder

LOCATION OF POINT: D–16 (right hand only); E–16 (right hand), E–19 (?); F–16 (right hand only)

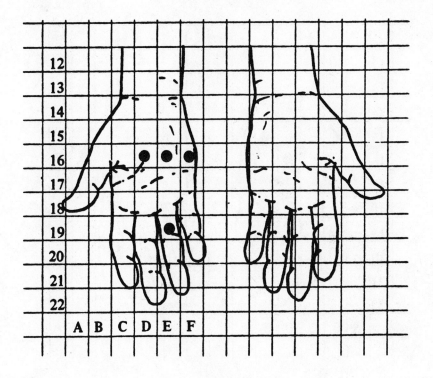

NAME OF HAND POINT: Gastrointestinal

LOCATION OF POINT: D-16; E-15

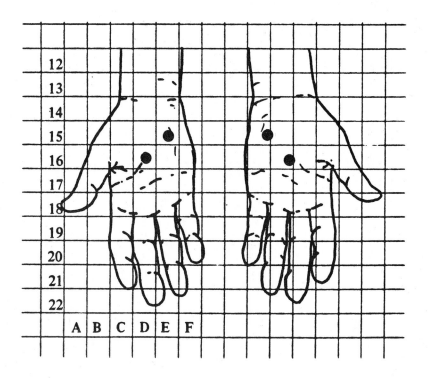

NAME OF HAND POINT: Head

LOCATION OF POINT: B-5

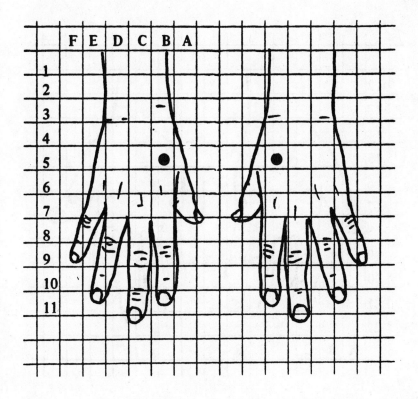

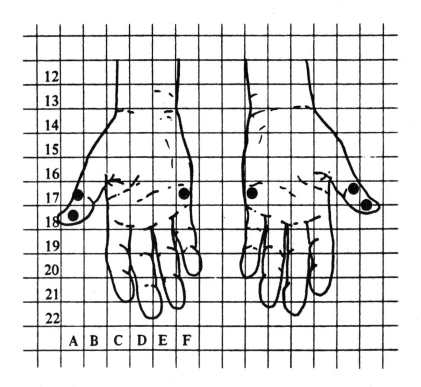

NAME OF HAND POINT: Heart

LOCATION OF POINT: C-15, 17 (left hand only); D-17 (left hand only), D-21; E-16 (left hand); F-15, 16, 17

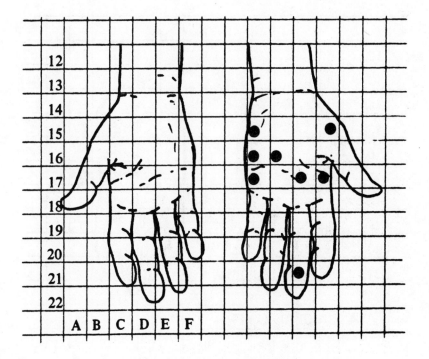

NAME OF HAND POINT: Heel

LOCATION OF POINT: D-14

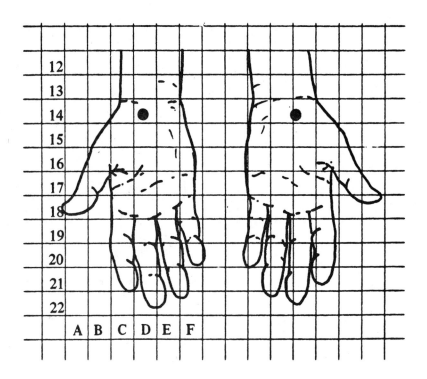

NAME OF HAND POINT: Hip

LOCATION OF POINT: E-14; F-14

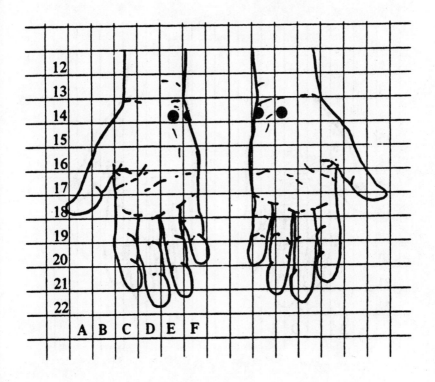

NAME OF HAND POINT: Hypothalamus

LOCATION OF POINT: A-17

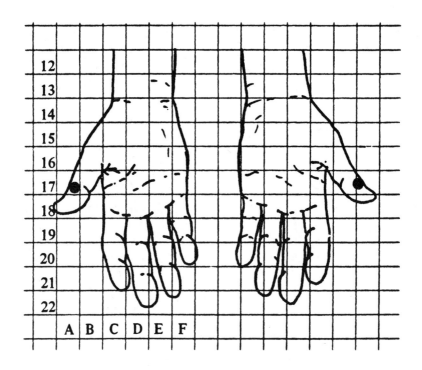

NAME OF HAND POINT: Ileo-cecum

LOCATION OF POINT: E-15 (right hand only)

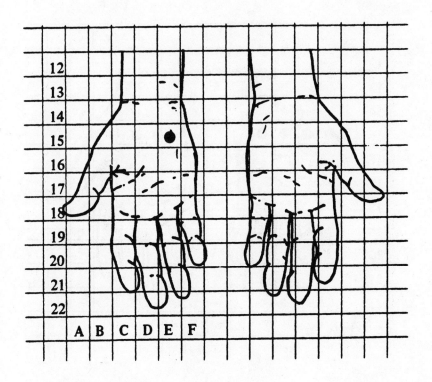

NAME OF HAND POINT: Intestine, small

LOCATION OF POINT: B-15; C-15, 19; D-15; E-15

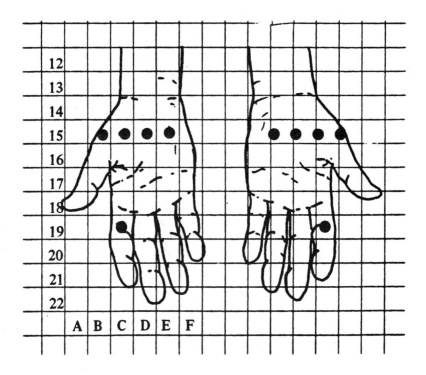

NAME OF HAND POINT: Kidneys

LOCATION OF POINT: D-17; E-15, 16, 17

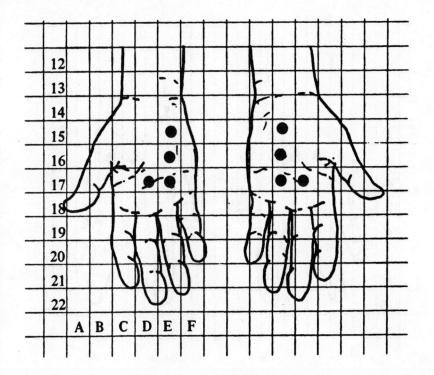

NAME OF HAND POINT: Leg

LOCATION OF POINT: C-5; D-5

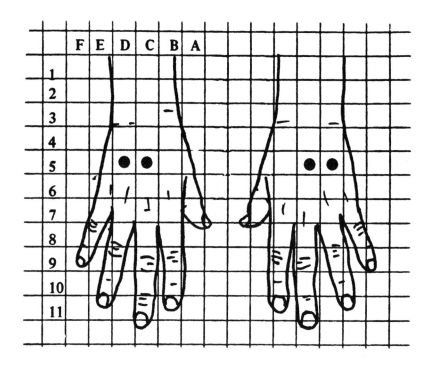

NAME OF HAND POINT: Liver

LOCATION OF POINT: D-16 (right side only); E-16 (right side), E-17, 19; F-16 (right side only), F-17

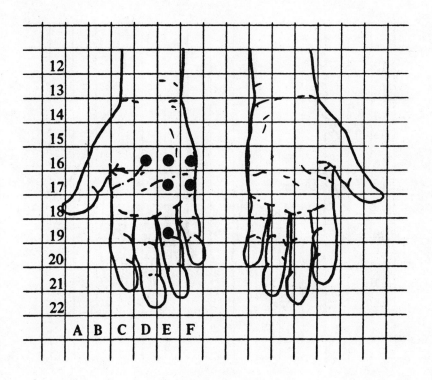

NAME OF HAND POINT: Lungs

LOCATION OF POINT: C-17; D-16, 17, 18; E-17

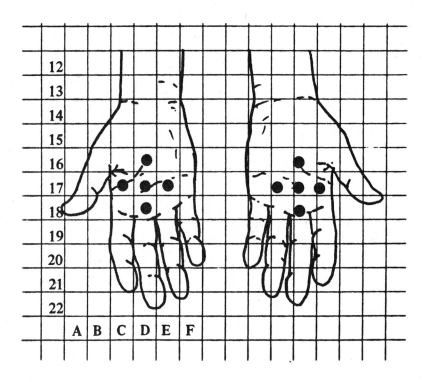

NAME OF HAND POINT: Mastoid

LOCATION OF POINT: F-17

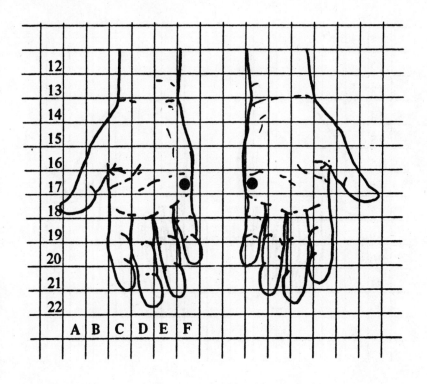

NAME OF HAND POINT: Mental powers,
facilities

LOCATION OF POINT: A-18; B-18

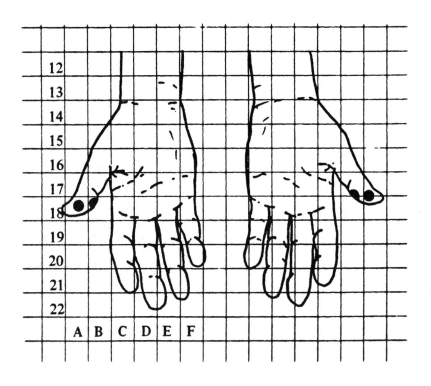

NAME OF HAND POINT: Mouth

LOCATION OF POINT: D-18

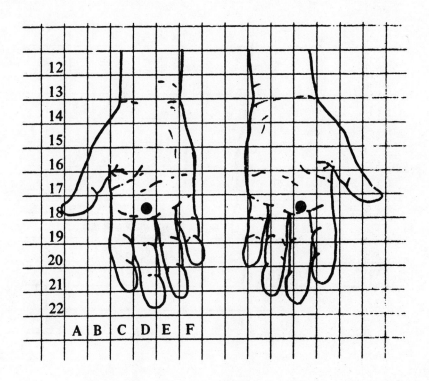

NAME OF HAND POINT: Muscles; muscular
    strength

LOCATION OF POINT: C-15, 16, 19, 20, 21; D-19, 20, 21,
    22

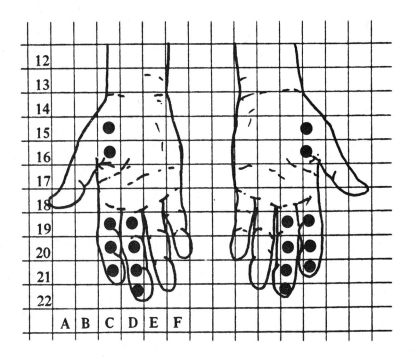

NAME OF HAND POINT: Neck

LOCATION OF POINT: B-7; C-7

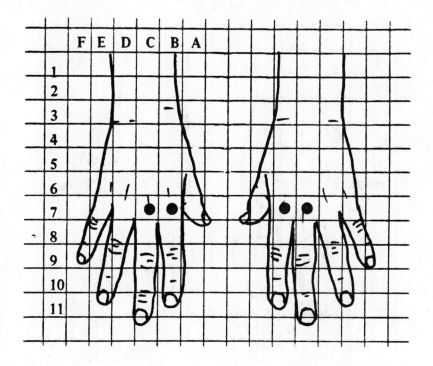

NAME OF HAND POINT: Neck continued...

LOCATION OF POINT: A-17; B-15, 16, 17

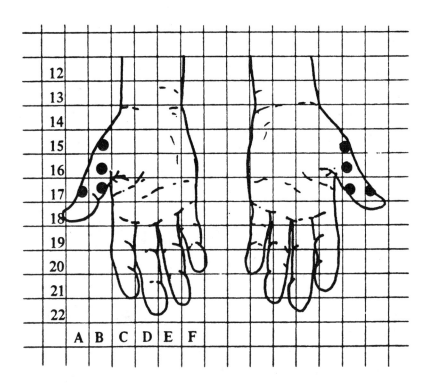

NAME OF HAND POINT: Nerves

LOCATION OF POINT: A-17, 18; B-15, 16, 17, 18; C-19, 20, 21; D-19, 20, 21, 22

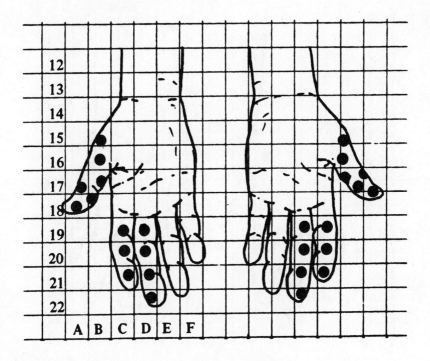

NAME OF HAND POINT: Nose

LOCATION OF POINT: B-5

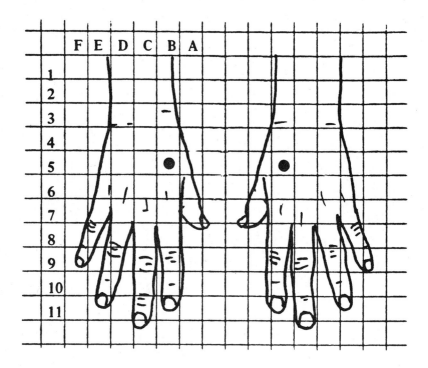

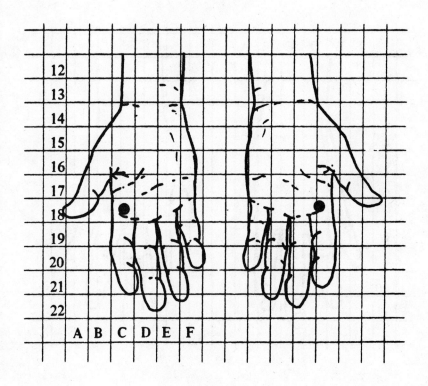

NAME OF HAND POINT: Occiput (back of head)

LOCATION OF POINT: E-7; F-7

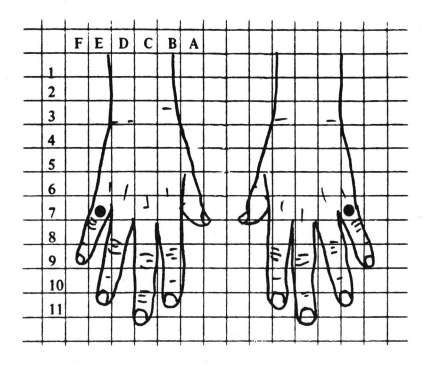

NAME OF HAND POINT: Ovary

LOCATION OF POINT: E-13, 14

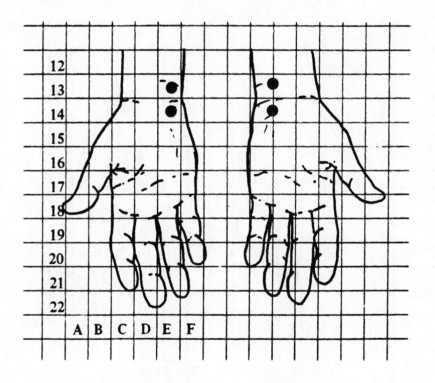

NAME OF HAND POINT: Pancreas

LOCATION OF POINT: D-16 (left hand only), D-17; E-16, 17, E-20, 21 (left hand only)

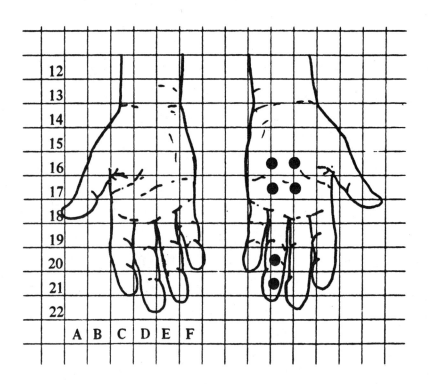

NAME OF HAND POINT: Parotid gland

LOCATION OF POINT: F-18

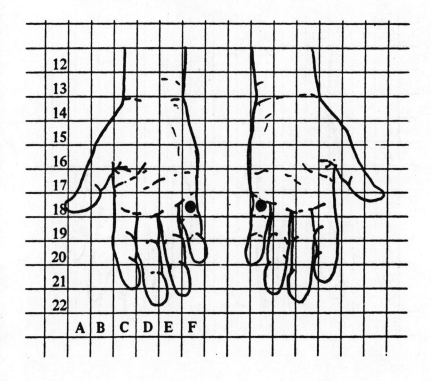

NAME OF HAND POINT: Perineum

LOCATION OF POINT: E-8

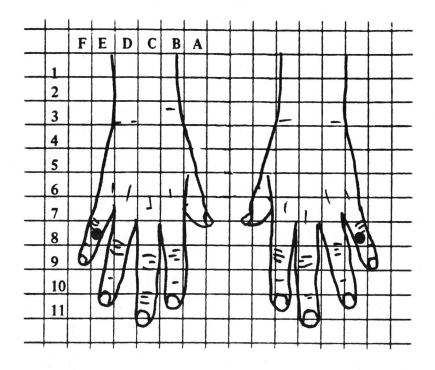

NAME OF HAND POINT: Pineal gland

LOCATION OF POINT: A-18

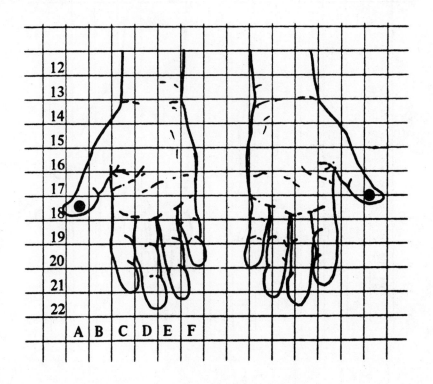

NAME OF HAND POINT: Pituitary gland

LOCATION OF POINT: A-18

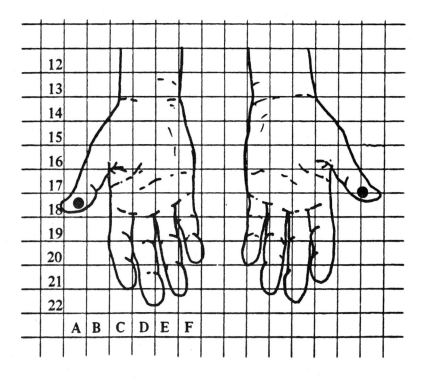

NAME OF HAND POINT: Prostate

LOCATION OF POINT: C-13

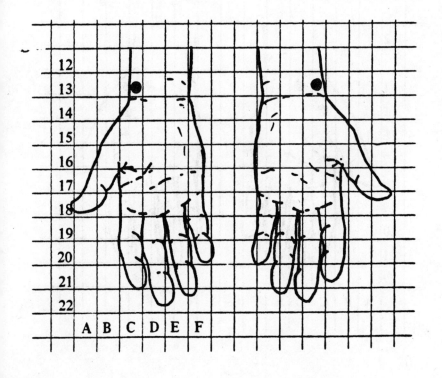

NAME OF HAND POINT: Rectum

LOCATION OF POINT: C-14, 15; D-14

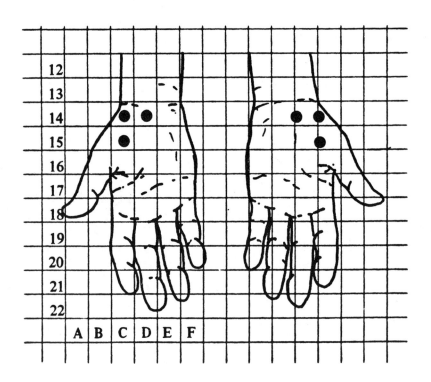

NAME OF HAND POINT: Sciatic nerve

LOCATION OF POINT: D-6, 7

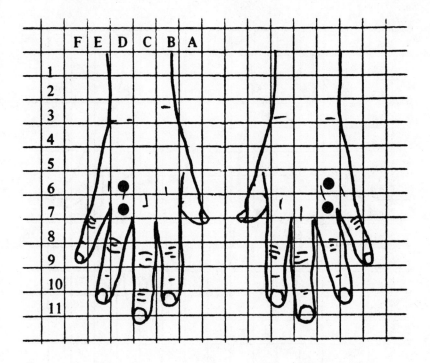

NAME OF HAND POINT: Sex organs

LOCATION OF POINT: C-13; D-14; E-14

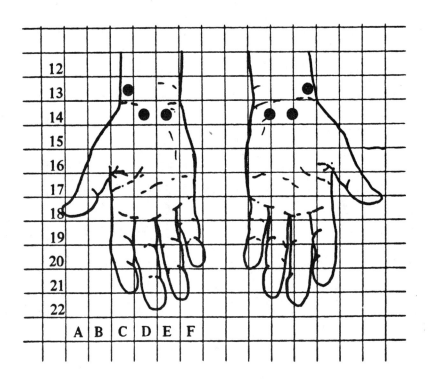

NAME OF HAND POINT: Shoulder

LOCATION OF POINT: B-7

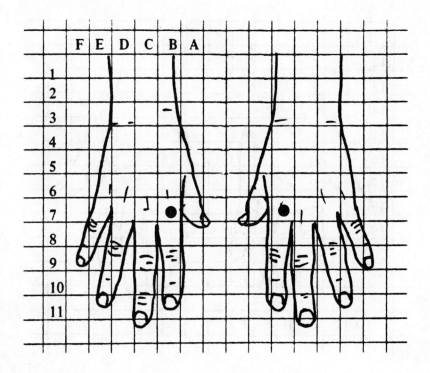

NAME OF HAND POINT: Shoulder continued...

LOCATION OF POINT: F-15

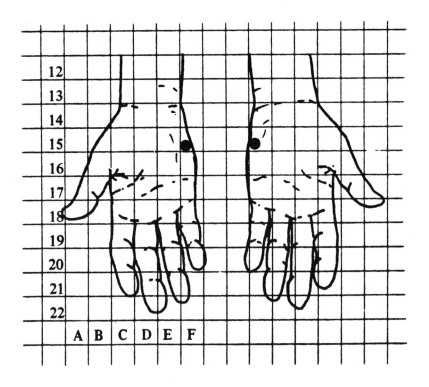

NAME OF HAND POINT: Sigmoid colon, flexure

LOCATION OF POINT: E-14 (left hand only)

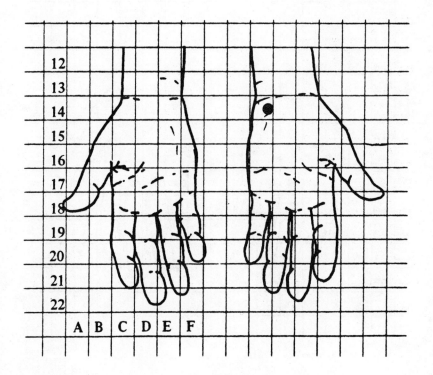

NAME OF HAND POINT: Sinuses

LOCATION OF POINT: C-18; D-18; E-18; F-18

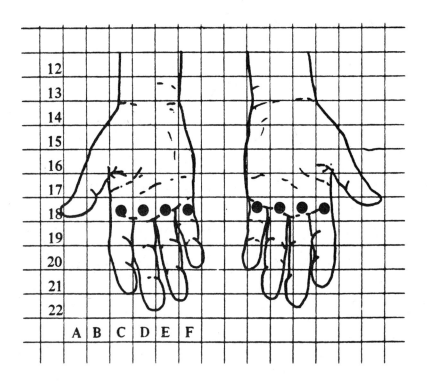

NAME OF HAND POINT: Solar plexus

LOCATION OF POINT: C-17

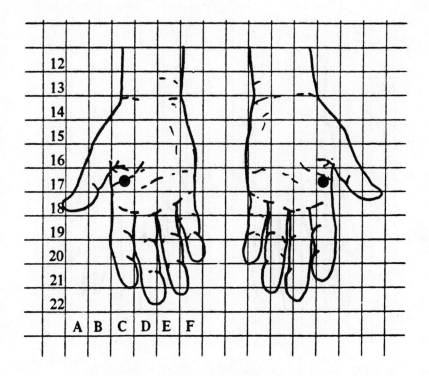

NAME OF HAND POINT: Spinal cord

LOCATION OF POINT: E-6

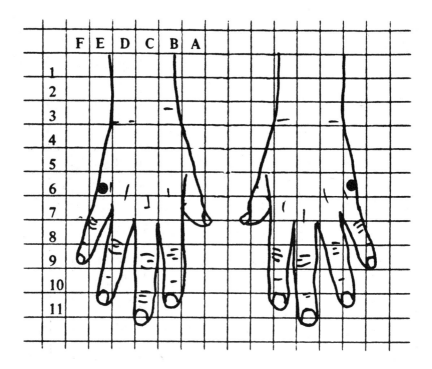

NAME OF HAND POINT: Spinal cord continued...

LOCATION OF POINT: C-14, 15, 16, 17

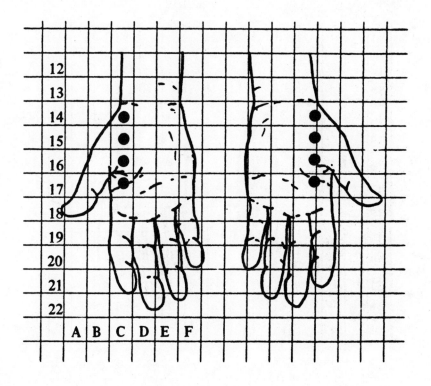

NAME OF HAND POINT: Spleen

LOCATION OF POINT: D-16 (left hand only); E-15, **16** (left hand only), E-20, 21 (left hand ?); F-15 (left hand only)

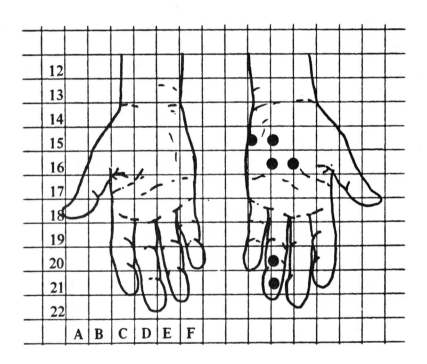

NAME OF HAND POINT: Stomach

LOCATION OF POINT: C-16, 17; D-16

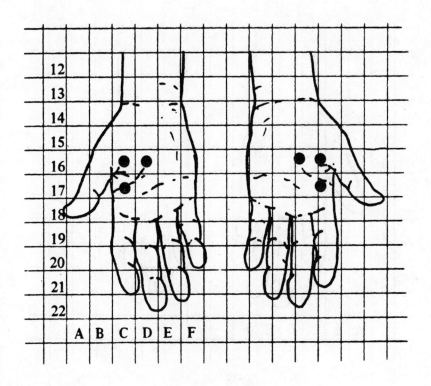

NAME OF HAND POINT: Testicles

LOCATION OF POINT: E-13

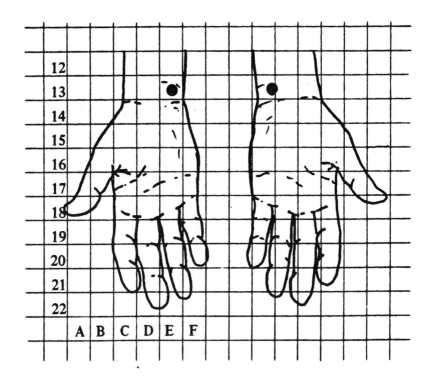

NAME OF HAND POINT: Throat

LOCATION OF POINT: C-7; D-7

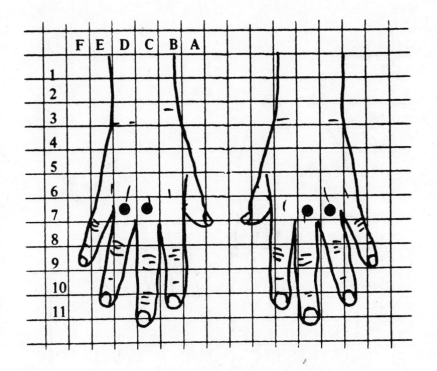

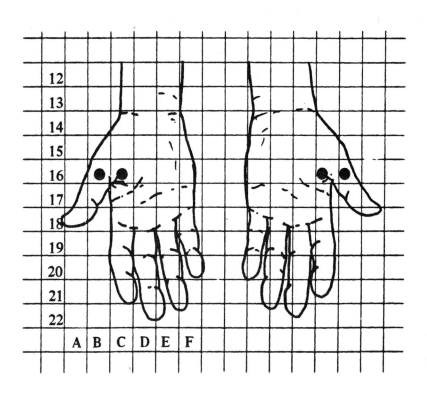

NAME OF HAND POINT: Thymus

LOCATION OF POINT: C-18; D-17, 18

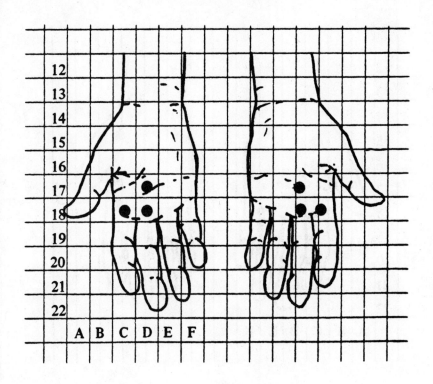

NAME OF HAND POINT: Thyroid and parathyroid

LOCATION OF POINT: C-15, 16, 18

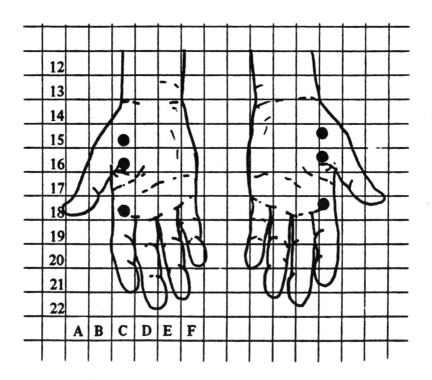

NAME OF HAND POINT: Tonsils

LOCATION OF POINT: C-17, 18

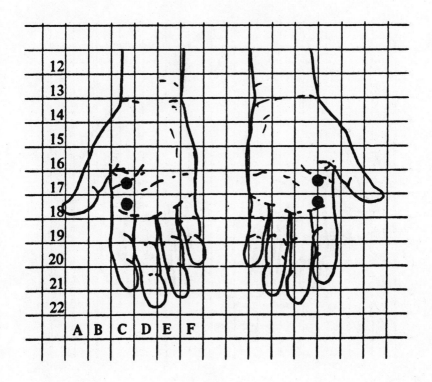

NAME OF HAND POINT: Tooth; teeth

LOCATION OF POINT: D–18

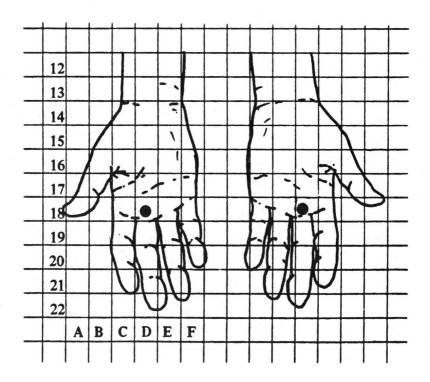

NAME OF HAND POINT: Uterus

LOCATION OF POINT: C-13

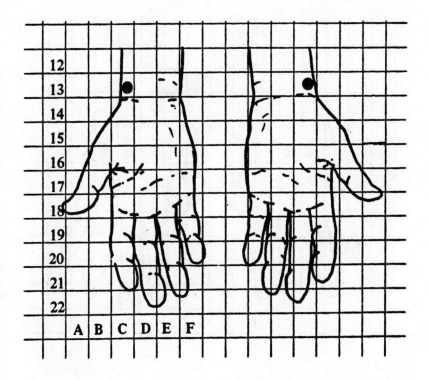

NAME OF HAND POINT: Vertebrae

LOCATION OF POINT: C-5; D-5

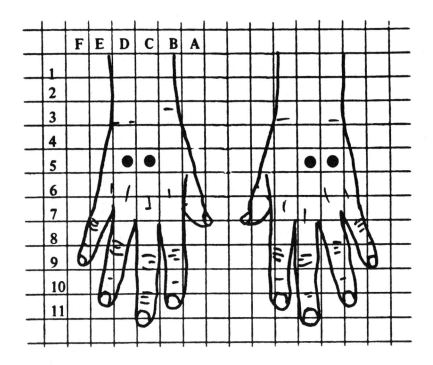

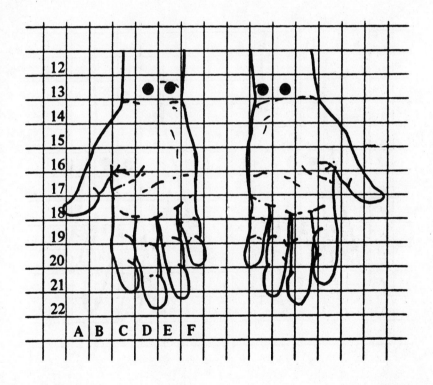

NAME OF HAND POINT: Waist

LOCATION OF POINT: C-5; D-5

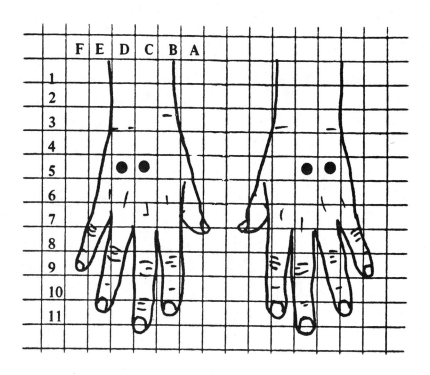

NAME OF HAND POINT: Wrist

LOCATION OF POINT: C-4

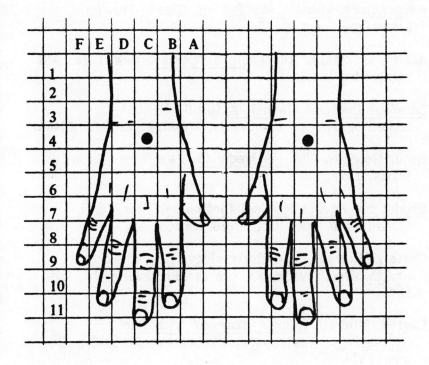

BIBLIOGRAPHY

The following publications have been helpful to the author and/or will be of interest for further studies by the reader.

Acupuncture Anaesthesia. Peking, China: Foreign Languages Press, 1972.

Austin, Dr. Mary. Acupuncture Therapy. New York: ASI Publishers, Inc. 1972.

Barefoot Doctor's Manual, A (N.I.H. 75-695) Superintendant of Documents, Washington, D.C. 20402.

Beau, Georges. Chinese Medicine. New York: Avon Books, 1972.

Blakiston's Pocket Medical Dictionary. New York: McGraw-Hill Book Co., third edition, 1972.

Carter, Mildred. Hand Reflexology: Key to Perfect Health. West Nyack, NY: Parker Publishing Co., Inc., 1975.

Carter, Mildred. Helping Yourself With Foot Reflexology. West Nyack, NY: Parker Publishing Co., Inc., 1974.

Cerney, J. V., A.B., D.M., D.P.M. Acupuncture Without Needles. West Nyack, NY: Parker Publishing Co., Inc., 1974.

Chan, Pedro, Finger Acupressure. Los Angeles: Price/Stern/Sloan Publishers, 1974

Chan, Pedro. Wonders of Chinese Acupuncture. Alhambra, CA: Borden Publishing Co., 1973.

Dale, Ralph A., Ph.D., Ed.D. Acupuncture with Your Fingers. Surfside, FL: Dialectic Press, P.O. Box 6622, 1980.

Dale, Ralph A., Ph.D., Ed.D. Acupuncture in Physical Therapy. Surfside, FL: Dialectic Press, 1981.

Dale, Ralph A., Ph.D., Ed.D. Microacupuncture Systems (books One and Two). Surfside, FL: Dialectic Press, 1981.

Duke, Marc. Acupuncture. New York: Pyramid Books, 1972.

Hashimoto, Mme. Dr. M. Japanese Acupuncture. 91 St. Martins Lane, London W.C.2, England: Thorson's Publishers, Ltd., 1962.

Houston, F.M., D.C. The Healing Benefits of Acupressure. New Canaan, CT.: Keats Publishing, Inc., 1974.

Huang, Helena L., Ph.D. (translator) Ear Acupuncture. Emmaus, PA: Rodale Press, 1974.

Ingham, Eunice D. Stories the Feet Can Tell. Rochester, NY: Eunice D. Ingham, Box 948, 1959.

Ingham, Eunice D. Stories the Feet Have Told.
Rochester, NY: Eunice D. Ingham, 1959.

Jain, K.K., M.D. The Amazing Story of Health Care in
China. Emmaus, PA: Rodale Press, 1973.

Kao, Frederick F., editor. The American Journal of
Chinese Medicine., Volumes I, II, III, through
number 3, July, 1975.

Kushi, Michio. Acupuncture, Ancient and Future
Worlds. Boston: East West Foundation, 1979.

Kushi, Michio. An Introduction to Oriental Diagnosis.
London: Red Moon Press; 12 Orpheus St., S.E.5, 1978.

Lavier, Dr. J. Points of Chinese Acupuncture
(translated, indexed, and adapted by Dr. Philip M.
Chancellor). Denington Estate, Wellingborough,
Northhamptonshire, England: Health Science Press,
second edition, 1974.

Lawson-Wood, D. & J. Acupuncture Handbook. England:
Health Science Press, second edition, 1973.

Lawson-Wood, D. & J. First Aid at Your Fingertips.
England: Health Science Press, 1963.

Lawson-Wood, D. & J. Five Elements of Acupuncture and
Chinese Massage. England: Health Science Press,
1966.

Lawson-Wood, D. & J. Judo Revival Points, Athletes'
Points and Posture. England: Health Science Press,
1960.

Lawson-Wood, D. & J. The Incredible Healing Needles. England: Health Science Press, 1974.

Lu, Henry, Ph.D. Chinese Acupressure. Vancouver, B.C., V6M 4G1, Canada: Academy of Oriental Heritage, P.O. Box 35057, Station E, 1977.

Lu, Henry, Ph.D. Introduction to Chinese Manipulative Therapy. Vancouver: Academy of Oriental Heritage, 1978.

Lu, Henry, Ph.D. Physicians' Guide to Dr. Lu's Chinese Diagnosis and Treatment Charts. Vancouver: Academy of Oriental Heritage, 1977.

Manaka, Dr.Y., and Urquhart, Dr.I.A. Chinese Massage. San Francisco: Japan Publications Trading Co., 1973.

Mann, Felix, M.B. Acupuncture, the Ancient Chinese Art of Healing. London: Wm. Heinemann Medical Books, Ltd., second edition, 1972.

Mann, Felix, M.B. Acupuncture, the Ancient Chinese Art of Healing and How It Works Scientifically. New York: Vintage Books (division of Random House)., 1973.

Mann, Felix, M.B. Acupuncture, Cure of Many Diseases. London: Wm. Heinemann Medical Books, Ltd., 1971.

Mann, Felix, M.B. The Treatment of Disease by Acupuncture. London: Wm. Heinemann Medical Books, Ltd., 1971.

Masunaga, Shizuto. Zen Shiatsu. San Francisco: Japan Publications Trading Co., 1977.

Matsumoto, Teruo, M.D., Ph.D., F.A.C.S. Acupuncture for Physicians. Springfield, IL: Charles C. Thomas, Publishers, 1974.

Merck Manual of Diagnosis and Therapy, The. Rahway, NJ: Merck & Co., Inc. eleventh edition, 1966.

McGarey, Wm. A., M.D. Acupuncture and Body Energies. Phoenix, AR: Gabriel Press, 1974.

Moss, Dr. Louis. Acupuncture and You. London: 2 All Saints St., N.1.: Elek Books, 1964.

Namikoshi, Tokujiro. Shiatsu: Health and Vitality at Your Fingertips. San Francisco: Japan Publications Trading Co., 1969.

Namikolshi, Toru. Shiatsu Therapy: Theory and Practice. San Francisco: Japan Publications Trading Co., 1977.

Ohashi, Wataru. Do-it-yourself Shiatsu. San Francisco: Japan Publications Trading Co., 1976.

Ohsawa, George. Acupuncture and the Philosophy of the Far East. Los Angeles: Tao Books, 1971.

Ohsawa, George. The Unique Principle. San Francisco: Geo. Ohsawa Macrobiotic Foundations, Inc., 1973.

Outline of Chinese Acupuncture, An. Peking: Foreign Languages Press, 1975.

Palos, Stephan. The Chinese Art of Healing. New York: Bantam Books, 1972.

Saran, Steve. Body Messages (charts I and II). Boulder, CO: Aslan Enterprises, 1979.

Saran, Steve. Reflexology (chart). Boulder, CO: Aslan Enterprises, 1979.

Saran, Steve. Unique Principle, The (chart). Boulder, CO: Aslan Enterprises, 1979.

Segal, Maybelle, R.N., R.D., N.D., I.D. Reflexology. North Hollywood, CA: Melvin Powers/Wilshire Book Company, 1976.

Serizawa, Katsusuke, Prof., M.D. Massage, the Oriental Method. San Francison: Japan Trading Co., 1972.

Serizawa, Katsusuke, Prof., M.D. Tsubo: Vital Points for Oriental Therapy: San Francisco: Japan Publications Trading Co., 1976.

Shultz, William. Shiatsu: Japanese Finger Pressure Therapy. New York: Bell Publishing Co., 1976.

Silverstein, M.E., et al. Acupuncturre and Moxibustion (prepared by the Dept. of Health, Ho Pei Providence, China). New York: Schocken Books, Inc., 1975.

Stiefvater, Dr. Eric H. What is Acupuncture? How Does It Work? England: Health Science Press, 1971.

Teeguarden, Iona. Acupressure Way of Health: Jin Shin Do. San Francisco: Japan Publications Trading Co., 1978.

Thakkur, Chandrashekhar, Dr. Ayurveda: The Indian Art and Science of Medicine. New York: ASI Publishers, 1974.

Thie, John F., D.C. Touch for Health. Santa Monica, CA: DeVorss and Co., Publishers, 1973.

Tibetan Medicine. Berkeley, CA: University of
California Press, 1976.

Toguchi, Masaru. The Complete Guide to Acupuncture.
New York: Frederick Fell Publishers, Inc., 1974.

Veith, Ilza (translated and introduced by). The Yellow
Emperor's Classic of Internal Medicine (Huang Ti Nei
Ching Su Wen). Berkely, CA: University of California
Press, 1972.

Wallnofer, Heinrich, and Von Rottauscher, Anna.
Chinese Folk Medicine. New York: New American
Library, Inc., 1972.

Warren, Frank Z., M.D. Freedom From Pain Through
Acupressure. New York: Frederick Fell Publishers,
1976.

Wei-P'ing, Dr. Wu. Chinese Acupuncture. England:
Health Science Press, 1962.

Wilner, R. E., M.D. Acupuncture Desk Reference. North
Miami Beach, FL: Medical Diagnostic Institute, 1974.

Wilner, R. E., M.D. Confidential Report: Acupressure.
Miami Beach, FL: Medical Diagnostic Institute, 1979.

Yamamoto, Shizuko. Barefoot Shiatsu. San Francisco:
Japan Publications Trading Co., 1979.

Yanagiya, S. Prof., Dr. One-Needle Acupuncture.
London: The Acupuncture Association.

COLOPHON:

The copy for this book was first entered into a Radio Shack TRS-80 Model II® computer using SCRIPSIT 2.0® software. After a number of printouts and editings, it was finally finished on a Radio Shack Daisy Wheel II® printer, set in Bold PS® typeface. It was then illustrated and delivered to Cash Printing, in Davie, FL, for printing and binding.

It was one of the 14 books written and produced simultaneously, during the spring and early summer of 1982, at Falkynor Farm, headquarters of Falkynor Books.

The advent of the micro-computer has radically altered the nature of many things — including that of publishing. Computerized publishing has heralded an "information explosion," bringing with it new challenges in book concept and design. We hope that our answer to those challenges — this book and its relatively unique format — will meet with your approval.